TOO
YOUNG FOR
CANCER

TOO YOUNG FOR CANCER

One Woman's Battle for a Diagnosis and a Fighting Chance

Katie Coleman

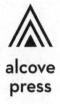

alcove
press

Published in the United States by Alcove Press, an imprint of The Quick Brown Fox & Company LLC.

Alcove Press and its logo are trademarks of The Quick Brown Fox & Company LLC.

Library of Congress Catalog-in-Publication data available upon request.

ISBN (hardcover): 978-1-63910-944-9
ISBN (ebook): 978-1-63910-945-6

Cover design by Heather VenHuizen

Printed in the United States.

www.alcovepress.com

Alcove Press
34 West 27th St., 10th Floor
New York, NY 10001

First Edition: November 2024

10 9 8 7 6 5 4 3 2 1

To my husband,
who stood by me every step of the way.
To the team of doctors who took a chance
on me, fostered my learning, and walked
with me through miles of uncertainty.
And to the many patients who supported
me through my darkest days.
Without you, I wouldn't have a story to tell.

Foreword

How do you deal with a cancer that is not even supposed to exist? This was the challenge Katie Coleman faced at just twenty-nine years old. She introduces her story by sharing vivid snapshots of her life: growing up in a small, one-stoplight town in Utah, relocating to Texas, then moving back to Utah to find true love after a divorce, all while forging a career in software engineering. Katie's narrative is marked by a candor and introspection that deeply resonate. Which makes it hit even harder when we find out about her potentially terminal diagnosis.

Katie has a knack for capturing the essence of each moment and interaction along her journey. Shortly after her diagnosis, she recounts attending a webinar I presented in 2021 on rare forms of kidney cancer. I looked again at that talk's busy slides and can attest that Katie perfectly summarized its key messages. That is remarkable for someone whose life has just been upended by a cancer diagnosis! Thanks to this skill, other patients today learn from Katie how to advocate for themselves and overcome relentless setbacks. Among the many pearls she shares with us, the observation that "strength isn't the absence of fear but instead a product of persevering through it" profoundly resonates. From Katie's story, we clinicians also acquire a deeper insight into the bewildering and truly frightening nature of a cancer diagnosis as well as the profound effect that even the smallest acts of empathy can achieve.

Katie's experience is now prompting us to revise our textbooks to include cases like hers and outline strategies to manage them. To navigate unprecedented challenges, we first need to remind ourselves, what does it mean for something to be "common"? The Bayesian system of inference used in many scientific applications stipulates that things are only similar to the extent that differences are overlooked. The regularities we see in nature are simply a projection of our minds. Nothing is ever truly repeated. Every single patient carries the most unique disease: it belongs to them alone. We artificially create patterns by ignoring the details. Take snowflakes, for instance: each exhibits sixfold symmetry, with crystals extending in six directions. Yet the old adage that no two snowflakes are alike holds true. The symmetry emerges only when we disregard the unique variations present in each snowflake.

Armed with this understanding, we can flip the narrative and create a tractable question: what are the details we need to ignore to find symmetries between Katie's disease and other cancers? This enables us to formulate plausible strategies for determining which treatments to pursue and which to avoid. For example, while immunotherapy has undoubtedly benefited numerous patients with cancer, there is considerable evidence suggesting that in tumors akin to Katie's, it may not offer help and could instead produce only adverse side effects.

It takes a village to develop and execute these strategies. Katie diligently assembled a care team from across the country with whom she felt at ease. This collaborative approach, along with the invaluable lessons we continually learn from our patients, stands as one of the most rewarding elements of practicing medicine.

—Pavlos Msaouel, MD, PhD

— 1 —

I feel like my life has just begun. I found a true, healthy and deep love. All I want to do is spend my life with him and build our lives together.
—Journal entry, December 30, 2020,
the day before I was diagnosed

I LET OUT A deep exhale as the car rolled to a stop in front of the emergency room entrance. The large tents erected at the front of the building reminded me of a scene from a postapocalyptic movie. It was New Year's Eve 2020, and with the pandemic in full swing, we'd heard family might not be allowed inside with patients due to COVID-19 protocols. The thought of waiting alone in an ER with nothing more the company of my racing thoughts sounded like a nightmare, but we knew we didn't have much choice. I looked over at my husband Brian one final time before reaching for the door.

"You've got this. Everything's going to be okay," he encouraged, giving me a kiss and squeezing my hand as I reluctantly unbuckled. "And keep me updated," he reminded as I squeezed his hand back just before stepping out and gently swinging the door shut.

As I made my way to the entrance, my mind raced through the worst possible scenarios of what the mass in my stomach could be. My eyes began to fill with tears. I'd felt like something was off with my body for years, but no one else seemed to agree. I was terrified of what they might find but equally scared of leaving once again with unanswered questions from a roomful of people who didn't believe me.

As I approached the tent, a nurse in full personal protective equipment (PPE) greeted me. As she asked what I'd arrived for, I instantly froze, unsure what to say as I retraced my steps through the downward spiral that'd led me here—one that can be visibly tracked through my internet browsing history in the days leading up to my arrival.

A broad search for "abdominal mass" would eventually turn into "symptoms of liver tumors," and hours later, I found myself in bed watching a YouTube video over my shoulder while trying to self-examine and palpate my abdomen for an enlarged liver. I knocked my phone from the nightstand again and again while I poked and prodded at my stomach with each new set of instructions. I was deep down the rabbit hole, and there was no turning back. I lost myself for hours spiraling through the worst possible scenarios before calling it a night with one last search of the evening for "soothing meditation music," a clear attempt to purge the panic I'd brought upon myself. A process I'd start all over again the next day.

The following morning, I woke and slid my hand over the upper part of my stomach, where I'd felt the firmness beneath my ribs the night before. I couldn't feel it now. *Is this all in my head?* Continuing the search, I rolled to my left side and pressed in. Nothing. Then, to the right. I felt fullness and discomfort but still no hardness or mass.

I got out of bed and made my way into the bathroom, poking at and feeling around my stomach with one hand while I brushed my teeth with the other. As soon as I caught the edge of it again, I paused, held perfectly still, and quickly called Brian over to look before I lost it again.

"That lump in my stomach is there again. Can you feel it?" I asked as I reached for his hand.

"Feel what?" he replied, confused.

"That hardness under my ribs, it's right here. Look, feel." I pulled him over and guided his hand to where mine was.

"Okay . . . what exactly am I supposed to be feeling?" he asked, the skepticism clear in his voice.

"I don't know. It's hard, like harder than the other side, and the edge is kind of round. Can't you feel it?" I insisted.

"No, I just feel stomach. I don't know what I'm supposed to be feeling . . ." I could sense his impatience mounting. I'd caught him as he was heading down to begin work, and he wasn't in the mindset to entertain my latest hypochondriacal episode. Brian had been supportive through all my health issues. But none of my other symptoms had ever panned out to be anything other than anxiety, according to the doctors, and he seemed to be getting a little fatigued.

I decided to wait for him to go downstairs before making my way over to the full-length mirror in our closet for a better look. As I stood in front of the mirror, I sucked in, twisted to the side, crunched, and turned, trying to get a glimpse of the elusive protrusion. After several tries, I started to pick up on the specific combination of breath-holding, flexing, and sticking my stomach out in just the right manner that would expose the bump. When I got the combination just right, I could gently press in and slightly cup my hand around it. *What is this thing?*

While I'd never been able to cup my hand around it before, the firmness was something I'd identified a couple of years ago. Something I distinctly remembered, because whenever I'd start a new diet or get on a workout streak, I'd always compare my body in the mirror, searching for progress. Sucking in, twisting, and flexing—honestly, not too dissimilar to the contortion I'd just been making but for reasons far vainer.

During one of these comparisons, I'd found a firmness on my right side and remembered wondering if it could be little baby abs budding. I'd been overweight most of my life, and at 170 pounds on a short five-foot-one frame, I liked the idea of progress brewing beneath the weight I'd struggled to melt off. I mentally congratulated myself for a job well done, and while I hadn't been met with the same firmness on the other side, I figured it just might need a little extra effort and attention to catch up.

I reflected on that memory as I poked at it some more. I'd noticed the firmness before but didn't remember feeling any of the edges that I swore I could feel now. I didn't know what this was, but I knew it would eat at me until I found out.

While I tried to decide whether I should take a trip to an urgent care, my mom called. Although we'd had plenty of trying times during my adolescence, she'd morphed into my best friend and my first call in adulthood. We spoke daily, so this was just another Wednesday evening.

That night, I brought her up to speed on my recent doctor appointments and the new hardness I was feeling just beneath my ribs. She began rattling off ideas of what it might be. But the more I described what I had been feeling, the more the fear rushed in, and I felt myself starting to get choked up. My worries started building, and all the time I'd spent in doctors' offices asking if we could rule out cancer finally caught up to me. I admitted, "I don't know what's wrong, but I'm worried it's cancer, and we've caught it too late, that it's stage four and has already gone to my liver."

Words that had been prompted by a spiraling Google search but still haunt me to this day, given the predicament I'd find myself in just a few hours later.

As we wrapped up the conversation, I looked up urgent care centers around me. It was getting late, and the next day was New Year's Eve. At eight PM, many of the urgent cares had already closed, but there was one open down the road, about fifteen miles from where we lived, closing in thirty minutes. With no time to second-guess myself, I went in.

As I arrived, the parking lot was well lit but empty. It was clear I was going to be the last patient for the evening. Walking into an urgent care ten minutes before closing felt like walking into a restaurant as they were stacking chairs and sweeping tables. I was convinced everyone would be annoyed.

As I made it to the counter to check in, I could feel my heart racing as I apologized for arriving so late. The young woman at the desk could clearly sense my anxiety and assured me it was okay before asking what had brought me in. What had led me to that moment felt like a culmination of far more than I could communicate in a single sentence. "I've started to feel a hardness just beneath my ribs," I fumbled out, breaking eye contact and gazing off to the corner of the building I wished I could disappear to.

I hadn't had the best relationship with the medical system. Over the past few years, I'd found myself in the ER twice and in countless doctors' offices in pursuit of answers to explain my symptoms. I'd never left with a diagnosis or answers to why I felt so off but rather just a new anxiety disorder added to my chart and an overwhelming sense of guilt and shame that I'd wasted everyone's time. Worried this evening would follow the same path, I averted my gaze to save myself from the judgment I was sure would be coming my way.

But instead of judgment, I noticed the woman's eyes soften as I was met with compassion. "Well, let's make sure we get you back to get it looked at. Are you in any pain?" I'd been feeling a mild ache for several days, but it was difficult to pinpoint, and it was so dull that it often made me wonder if maybe it was all in my head. I told her about it anyways as I passed my license and insurance under the plexiglass barrier. A few clicks, taps, and a quick scan later, she passed them back. "Okay, have a seat over there, and we'll call you soon. We don't have anyone waiting, so it should be quick."

I looked around the lobby while waiting to be called back. The building was new, with large windows and an open concept, a design I'd become familiar with from other clinics I'd visited. During the day, the open concept provided a welcome distraction from the wait, allowing me to watch the hustle and bustle of people making their way to their appointments or the health care workers mingling in the hallway. But as the last patient in for the night, tonight it looked much different. The halls were empty, and the building was cold and quiet, leaving me alone with my worries and all the what-ifs. Thankfully, it wasn't long until a nurse appeared in the doorway to call me back, and we made our way to a room.

As she wrapped the blood pressure cuff around my arm and placed the pulse ox on my finger, I watched her facial expression as she caught my heart rate. "One twenty-two. Are you nervous?" I'd had a rapid heart rate (tachycardia) for a while now and was used to this reaction. Before I'd been medicated for it, it was normal for me to clock in at 145 to 165 bpm (beats per minute), so 122 felt pretty reasonable. A resting heart rate for adults, according to the American Heart Association, is typically between 60 and 100 bpm. The nurse had me take a few slow, deep breaths until we got it down to 113 and my blood pressure to 144/88 before logging it into the chart and letting me know someone would be in shortly to see me. My blood pressure had been high for a number of years; before being medicated, it'd often come in at around 150/110 when the standard range is 120/80. That, along with my high resting heart rate, was one of the symptoms I had been telling doctors about that were continually explained away by anxiety.

As the nurse left the room and the door rolled shut behind her, I could hear the voices of the staff down the hall discussing their plans for New Year's as they closed up for the evening. As the voices trailed off, I heard footsteps approaching my room before a man walked in and introduced himself as Casey, the nurse practitioner who would be taking care of me that evening. He was relaxed and unrushed as he asked what had brought me in. I told him about the dull ache coming and going in my upper right abdomen and the mass I'd recently discovered. He acknowledged my concerns, nodded slowly, then paused, waiting for me to continue.

I was so used to being rushed through appointments and having my symptoms explained away that I was caught off guard at first. *Wait, what else am I supposed to tell him? Do I let him know I've been Googling my symptoms all day? Or do I keep those details close to my chest so I don't leave here with another anxiety diagnosis added to my chart?* I wasn't used to being given time to fully detail all my symptoms. I'd usually start, then be cut off with the same leading questions that always pointed us back to anxiety. Was my job ever stressful, was I getting enough sleep? The fatigue, hair thinning, rapid heart rate, high blood pressure, weight loss—all bucketed the second I'd respond with any remotely confirmatory answer like, "I don't know, maybe, but . . . ?" Before I completed the sentence, everything would be tidied up in a bow. "Yeah, stress and anxiety can do that. Let's work on getting that under control for you, and I think you'll feel much better."

I'd leave the room feeling disheartened and unheard but also guilty and confused. I was bitter at them for not listening but felt guilty for being bitter at someone trying to help me. It wasn't uncommon for me to watch their body language soften as they watched a tear trickle from the corner of my eye, indicating how scared and frustrated I was by the lack of answers and resolution to my symptoms. In most appointments, my physicians never lacked compassion; they lacked time. I knew most of them wanted to help me, and they thought they were. Which was one of the most frustrating parts of it all.

I avoided eye contact as I continued, deciding to take the risk and share with Casey what had really led me to come in. "Honestly, I don't know what's wrong. But I've been looking up symptoms, and I'm a little worried about it being an enlarged liver. So I wanted to come in to get it looked at before the holiday."

I felt ashamed to admit I'd been Googling my symptoms. But as I looked up, I wasn't met with an ounce of judgment. Casey nodded once more, asked a few follow-up questions, then requested I hop up onto the table so he could look. As I lay back, he began poking and pushing against my abdomen in a similar fashion to what I'd seen on the YouTube video the night before. During his examination, I explained that I hadn't been able to feel it while lying down but that it was more noticeable when I was standing. So he had me stand back up to show him instead.

I positioned my stomach in just the right position and showed him where my hand cupped around it. He then examined the area himself. After palpating the mass and following up with a few questions, he acknowledged he was able to feel it too. He thought it could be an enlarged liver and suggested that I follow up with my primary care provider (PCP) or that I go to the ER to get it further evaluated.

After years of being dismissed by others, Casey was the first person ever to take me seriously. As we wrapped up, he asked if I had any final questions. I had a million, but I limited myself to a few more before thanking him for his time and patience—a thank-you that didn't feel adequate for how much I truly appreciated his attentiveness. In a single thirty-minute appointment, Casey had made me feel more heard than I'd felt in years.

As I walked out of the clinic and back to the car, I began mulling over whether I should head to the ER. I wasn't in a tremendous amount of pain, and besides the hardness in my abdomen, overall I felt okay. This didn't exactly *feel* like an emergency. I had already mentioned it to my PCP a day or two prior, and they hadn't seemed concerned, so that didn't feel like a viable option. With the pandemic in full swing, I'd heard about how full the hospitals were, and I didn't want to be a distraction if this turned out to be nothing. But I had a nagging feeling that something was wrong, so I took Casey's advice and decided to head to the ER.

As I stood at the entrance to the tent in front of the hospital, nerves shook my voice as I told the intake nurse that the urgent care had advised me to come in, and my hands trembled as I fumbled through my wallet for my insurance card. Her eyes softened with compassion as she noticed the tears in my eyes.

"It's okay, let's just get you inside," she replied, passing me a mask and ushering me into the tent for screening. Once I was cleared, she personally escorted me and my green wristband through the makeshift hallways to the main entrance. "You've got it from here," she encouraged, holding the door open and gently gesturing me inside.

I waited anxiously in the cold, near-empty lobby before being called back and greeted by a chaotic scene on the other side. Monitors beeped, nurses bustled to and from each room, and a handful of patients in hospital beds lined the hallways. The fast-paced yet organized frenzy reminded me of a busy intersection as I tried to keep up with the nurse escorting me back to a room. *Why do they always walk so fast?* My short little legs struggled to keep up.

Before I knew it, we'd reached our destination, and I got settled in, awaiting the doctor's arrival. I'd even been informed by the friendly EMT starting my IV that Brian was allowed to come back and join me. I couldn't have been more relieved and instantly shot him a text, hoping he'd make it before the doctor arrived. But just as the EMT walked out of the room, a young doctor walked in.

He briefly introduced himself before inquiring about what'd brought me here. As I began explaining my symptoms and that the urgent care had sent me for a possible enlarged liver, the skepticism was evident on his face. He had me lie back as he began poking and prodding at my upper right abdomen just as Casey had done a few hours prior. "Any pain here?" he asked while pushing in, one hand layered over the other.

"No . . . ," I replied.

He adjusted locations and tried again. "What about this?"

"No, no pain," I confirmed.

And just like that, as quickly as he'd started the exam, he'd now finished and was removing his gloves as he shook his head. "Yeah, I don't know what they're talking about. I don't feel an enlarged liver," he confirmed, matter-of-factly, in a bit of a dismissive and rushed tone.

My cheeks flushed with embarrassment. *Great, he thinks I'm a hypochondriac. Am I just wasting everyone's time?* Making an attempt to sound far more casual and relaxed than I actually was, I told him that I felt it most while standing and that's how the nurse practitioner had felt it as well. He reaffirmed he hadn't found anything during the exam but suggested that if I really wanted it, he could order a CT scan just to be sure.

Even if he seemed a bit skeptical, this was far more than anyone else had been willing to explore. I was grateful he was willing to do a more thorough workup. So before he left the room, I took the time to pass along a sincere and honest thank-you, letting him know how much I appreciated him putting the order in just in case. He caught the tears forming behind my eyes as I shared the gratitude, causing him to pause just before he left the room. I felt his demeanor soften as he took a step back toward the bed. He placed a reassuring hand at the edge, letting me know we'd get everything checked out and he'd be back to check on me.

Since I was only twenty-nine, he had concerns about the radiation they might expose me to with a CT Scan, so he ended up placing an order for an ultrasound instead. Soon, the kind EMT who'd started my IV earlier reappeared. He casually spun a wheelchair at the foot of the bed as he gestured for me to hop in. I looked back at him, perplexed—my legs were fine; surely I could walk.

"The halls around here get a bit chilly, and we've got a ways to go. If you're feeling up to it, you can walk, or you can hitch a ride with me," he said, offering me a warm blanket. Already freezing from the glamorous hospital gown hanging off my shoulder and missing half its buttons, I bundled myself in the blanket and took him up on the offer.

As I entered the ultrasound room, a bubbly tech greeted me and politely asked how I was doing while I settled in and she prepped the equipment. Trying to make light of the situation through nervous laughter, I replied, "Oh, you know, been better."

She chuckled softly, spreading the warm gel across my stomach. "This shouldn't take long. We'll get you back to the room soon," she assured as she began the exam. Just as the pressure from the wand pressed in toward my ribs, the dynamic shifted in the room and I watched the emotion drain from her face. She lifted up, pivoted, and went back for a better look. Then another, and another, feverishly clicking away to capture images. My heart began to race. She'd found something.

After a few minutes of silence while she worked, she asked concernedly, "How's your blood pressure?"

"Uh . . . it's not great," I replied, followed by more nervous laughter. Except this time there was no laugh back.

Minutes felt like hours as she continued on, gliding the wand across my stomach, pushing and twisting it into position. With no response, I lay there in silence, torturing myself, wondering what could be on that screen. About halfway through the exam, she followed along the right side of my rib cage until my ribs met in the middle, pressed in, and let out a distressed sigh. She paused, trying to gather herself as she wiped a bead of sweat from her forehead.

I didn't know what she'd found but knew it couldn't be good. I watched her battle the emotions as she tried to mask her concern and couldn't help but wonder how often she found herself in this position: discovering something she knew would forever change the life of the person sitting in front of her. Knowing for a brief moment she was the only one in the world who knew but unable to say a word. I couldn't imagine the toll that must take.

After the ultrasound, I waited in the room with Brian, desperate to know what was going on. Over the next few hours, results and bad news slowly started flowing in. As if our room had suddenly become radioactive, the updates were fragmented and brief. Anyone who delivered news had one foot out the door, exiting as quickly as possible before we had time for questions, leaving us behind with what felt like a live bomb to disarm with nothing but a Google Search and trembling hands. In less than twenty-four hours, we'd gone from looking up the best neighborhood to raise a family in to Googling survival stats. *How did we end up here?*

— 2 —

If Grandma could find love several times in her final years,
then I certainly still had time.

Brian and I had known each other for only a little over a
year by the time we found ourselves in the ER that cold
December night. At the end of May 2019, I met Brian online,
and I fell head over heels for him almost instantly. But when
we first started dating, I often wondered if people would question how genuine our connection was if they knew the full
story. It's not exactly the type of story they write romance nov-
els about. A tale more fitting of a cancer memoir, apparently.

When Brian and I met, I had gone through a series of bad
breakups and had moved back to Utah after my grandma's
passing to be close to family and to help with the funeral. I
had previously been staying in an Airbnb camper on a small
winery just outside Temecula, California, shortly after the
abrupt end of a long relationship led me to sell my house in
Austin, Texas, and everything I owned to travel the West
Coast as a digital nomad. I hoped to find both myself and the
next place I'd call home along the way. But instead, after a few
short months, I found myself back in Utah in an old, dingy,
short-term rental that I could barely afford on my part-time
salary.

I'd grown up in a small, one-stoplight town about forty-five minutes outside Salt Lake City, then moved to Austin in my early twenties. The mountains back home were enchanting, and the diverse landscape between Northern and Southern Utah provided some of the most gorgeous views in the country. However, the winters were cold, and I found the seasonal depression that comes with the months of gloomy cloud cover suffocating. Though my grandma's passing had hit me hard, my move back to Utah was meant to be only a temporary detour to support my mom through her grief and to aid in her recovery from a minor surgery.

This was also reflected in my apartment, which was furnished with a frumpy, twenty-year-old couch and glass table from my mom's storage unit along with two wobbly chairs you had to carefully balance on to prevent them from collapsing. The only other furniture you'd find as you took a look around would be a cheap IKEA TV stand, which I'd somehow managed to assemble backwards, and a bed in a box I'd found on Walmart special that I'd rolled directly out onto the bedroom floor without a frame. Which is precisely where I found myself the night I matched on Bumble with Brian online.

That night, while I was cleaning and unpacking, I made a whiskey Coke in an attempt to cover up the grief of my grandma's passing and the breakup I'd gone through a few days prior. It felt like my life was falling apart and I was sitting by watching helplessly as everything crumbled around me. In a matter of months, I'd had two failed relationships, one of which had been several years long. I'd gone from being a homeowner to barely scraping by in a run-down apartment, had lost my grandmother, and was struggling as I worked to transition into a new career as a software engineer.

So, as I found places for the final items I had left to unpack, I began reminiscing over memories of my grandma, who I'd seen go through many life phases of her own over the years—one of which had been rediscovering and exploring the dating scene in her eighties. If Grandma could find love several times in her final years, then I certainly still had time.

During one of the last conversations I'd had with her, we'd swapped stories of our love lives while she was recovering from knee surgery. An experience that seems a bit crazy at face value—who swaps dating stories with their grandma?—but it's one that I look back on with great fondness. In the final years of her life, my grandma reentered the online dating scene. As she described to me each gentleman she encountered, she shared pictures, and a clear ranking system of her preferences began to emerge. The fellas with bad habits and "too much baggage" slowly made their way down the list, and those with great stories, adventures, and conversation quickly ascended to the top, with bonus points awarded to those who still had their teeth—a rare find for men in their eighties.

These connections resulted in her finding love several times in the span of just a few years. Each of them highlighted different sides to her personality and provided many stories and adventures that she cherished. Regardless of how the relationships ended, she described them each as their own encapsulated adventure. Her relationships were nothing to be ashamed of, forgotten about, or brushed under the rug. They were simply a new chapter in the choose-your-own-adventure game we call life.

Emboldened by Grandma and the whiskey Coke, I downloaded Bumble and let the adventure begin. I wasn't exactly in a rush to jump back into another relationship. After all, I'd just ended a short one a few days prior. But, curious about what the dating scene was like in Utah, I told myself I'd download the app and set up my profile just to check it out for the night.

The best part about online dating is you can do it from the mattress rolled out on your bedroom floor with unwashed hair, a stained T-shirt, and no makeup. Which is exactly how I found myself as I lay diagonally across my makeshift bed and began creating my profile. In my bio, I described myself as a short, outdoorsy-ish twenty-eight-year-old with shoulder-length, light-brown hair who had a small ten-pound, scruffy dog named Baxter. With the basics filled in, it was time to start swiping.

Within an hour, I'd swiped right on a few matches and begun striking up casual conversation. I continued to browse the app until I came across Brian's profile. A handsome thirty-year-old software engineer. His profile featured photos of him hiking and rock climbing and his adorable calico cat. Since I was in the middle of a shift in my career into software development, I figured we'd have a lot in common, so I swiped right and sent him a message.

We ended up messaging all night and into the early hours of the morning, getting to know each other through lighthearted conversations and flirtatious humor. I quickly became smitten in the days that followed as we messaged back and forth all day, every day, and as Brian tried to convince me we should meet in person. I was enjoying our conversation but still didn't feel ready to date and was self-conscious about my appearance. I'd chosen recent pictures for my profile, so it's not like I was catfishing, but I'd put on fifty pounds over the past few years and was worried he'd no longer be interested if he met me in person. So, every time he asked to meet up, I came up with an excuse and delayed our meeting for another day.

This continued for a couple of weeks until one evening, I finally built up the courage and asked if he'd like to meet for drinks. We settled on a bar down the street from his condo. I parked outside his place, and I texted him as I arrived. I nervously fixed my hair, checking my makeup again and again before taking a deep breath, reaching for the handle, and finally stepping out of the car. *This is it*, I thought as I made my way to the front of the building. *No turning back now.*

As he walked out and our eyes met for the first time, I felt the butterflies turn in my stomach as I tried to decode his expression. I was worried it might be disappointment, but I'd later learn it was the look of a nerdy guy with a limited dating history trying to contain his own nerves combined with the stoic expression he so naturally carries.

We made our way down to the bar for a couple of drinks and great conversation before eventually deciding to head back to his place as the bar emptied out for the night. Heading back to the house of a random stranger I met on the internet sounds like a great way to end up featured in a true-crime podcast, but this felt different. It felt like we'd known each other for years. So, as we closed our tab, I texted a friend to let them know who I was with and where I was going to be safe.

After a recent divorce, Brian had decided to start anew and had recently purchased a small one-bedroom condo from a family friend, moving in just a few weeks prior. As we walked through the door, we were greeted by Dora, his little calico, who I instantly crouched down to say hi to. She was the smallest, most adorable adult cat I'd ever seen. I silently added a few bonus points to the mental ranking I'd been keeping in my head and plopped down on the couch, where I'd hoped she'd join me as Brian stepped into the kitchen for drinks.

When he returned, he put two beers on the hand-me-down coffee table next to us, which we'd each take exactly one sip from and then leave untouched for the rest of the evening as we continued our conversation—meandering through all the topics you're not supposed to talk about on a first date. We found ourselves deep in dialogue about religion, politics, failed relationships, and everything in between until dawn, when the conversation was still flowing but our energy had dwindled. We both knew it was time to call it a night. We wrapped up the conversation, and I said goodbye to Dora with an adoring chin rub and made my way to the door.

As I reached for the handle, I paused to let Brian know I'd had a great night and hoped to see him again. He agreed from across the room as he nervously avoided eye contact. For a guy who'd seemed to be pretty into me as we were lost in conversation, he sure was keeping his distance. Was he really going to let me leave without even a hug? Our connection felt undeniable, but his body language made me wonder if I was completely off base. We stood awkwardly for a few seconds before I broke the ice. "Do I at least get a hug?" I asked, poking fun at the awkwardness we found ourselves in. He moved in for a quick embrace, and I headed out the door with a friendly goodbye.

The entire drive home, I questioned how I could have been so off about things. We'd spent several hours talking and sharing the deepest parts of our lives. Was I really getting friend-zoned on the first date? As I returned home with the sunrise breaking through my bedroom window, I crawled into my makeshift bed and turned out the lights just as I heard my phone vibrate. I glanced over to see a new message from Brian, making fun of himself and how nervous he'd been as we were saying our goodbyes. He shared how much he'd enjoyed the evening and that he'd been too nervous to go in for a hug, wanting to be respectful and worried it might be too forward for me on a first date. Which I only found more endearing. This man had plenty of wit and game behind a screen, but his nerdy nature shone through in person, which I fell even more in love with.

From that night forward, we were pretty much inseparable. I moved in within a few months. We were engaged by July 2020 and married just three months later, in October 2020, on my late grandma's birthday—our way of honoring her and our Bumble-inspired meeting.

After what had felt like a lifetime of heartbreak, I'd finally found my person, and I couldn't have been more excited about the life we had planned. Things had finally fallen into place, life was better than I could have ever imagined, and were in the full swing of the honeymoon phase when we received the news that would threaten our newly poured foundation and change both our lives forever.

— 3 —

*I'd be lying if I said I wasn't scared of what lies ahead of me
but I finally have a path and diagnosis to follow. Certainly
not one I'd ever want, but it was the cards I was dealt and
now we're going to learn to play them.*
                              —Instagram post, December 31, 2020

W HO'S GOING TO deliver the crushing cancer diagnosis
to the newlyweds in room five? I imagine this had to
have been one of the conversations occurring on the other side
of the door as Brian and I waited for the results of my final
scan. The two of us sat in silence, unaware that soon our new
vows would be tested while behind-the-scenes calls were being
made, referrals placed, and handoffs prepared.

We'd arrived at eleven PM, and as the clock rounded past
four AM, Brian and I were both beginning to doze off. We were
awakened by a new doctor who appeared in the doorway. As
he pulled up a stool next to the bed, he introduced himself as
Dr. Morgan. I took notice of the beaded bracelet he wore on
his wrist as he rested his hand gently on the bed, took a deep
breath, and softened his gaze to break the news. "The CT scan
we sent you for came back. We've found a large mass on your
right kidney and a couple lesions in your liver. We don't know
for sure, but we think it's likely renal cell carcinoma, a type of
kidney cancer."

My vision tunneled in as my heart rate, quickly escalating, began setting off alarms behind me. For years I had kept

asking doctors if we could rule out cancer in my pursuit of vague symptoms. I'd been terrified of this moment, and the catastrophic worrying had led me to imagine the delivery of this news probably a hundred times before. But now that it was actually happening, it was nothing like I'd imagined it would be. Despite my racing heart, *why did I feel so calm?* Brian squeezed my hand as I looked over my shoulder and watched him break into tears. That felt like the appropriate response here.

I shifted my gaze back to Dr. Morgan and asked in a calm and steady tone that surprised even me, "Is it terminal?"

I felt the emotion in his response. "We don't know. We'll need to run more tests and gather additional information, but we've already reached out to Huntsman Cancer Institute and have placed a referral to get you in as soon as possible. We may not have all the answers yet, but you have a whole team of doctors already working behind the scenes to figure this out."

Suddenly, I recognized the emotion that was washing over me. This wasn't grief. It was relief. It felt like I finally had an answer to why I'd been feeling off, and it wasn't all in my head. I wasn't surprised to hear something was wrong because I had *known* something was wrong; I just hadn't gotten anyone to take me seriously. But now we had undeniable proof, and for the first time, I was sitting across from a doctor who not only believed me but seemed to genuinely care. I knew this wouldn't be an easy road, but at least I no longer had to travel it alone.

As I thought about the appointments and memories that had led to this moment, the emotions finally caught up with me as I remembered the several doctors who had told me I was too young for cancer. The words looped in my head as I tried to make sense of it all before they found their way out without context.

"But other doctors told me I was too young for cancer." My voice broke, and the grief crashed over me as I finally began processing the news. My blood pressure, now climbing, set off more alarms as I looked at the monitor, concerned. Dr. Morgan reminded me I had just received some pretty distressing news. "That's a normal response; don't worry about those for now," he reassured me.

I focused again on the words circling in my head. "How could this happen? They told me I was too young for cancer . . . ," I said aloud again as my voice trailed off in disbelief. Dr. Morgan explained that we don't always know what causes cancer, empathetically apologized for the road that had led me here, and shared that this was personal for him, as his mom had battled with cancer as well. From the hint of sorrow in his voice, it sounded as if she might no longer be here. I wondered if this would be how people were going to talk about me one day too.

As he stood up to leave, I thanked him for answering my questions and being patient with me. I knew he likely had a busy ER to attend to. But he had brought a calming presence into the room and never once made us feel rushed, which I truly appreciated. I was grateful that it was him who delivered the news to me that day.

After he left the room, I turned to Brian and instantly apologized as we both began crying uncontrollably. I felt guilty, like I was robbing him of his future and the life we had planned together. He told me to stop; he wasn't going anywhere, and neither was I. I squeezed his hand as the door opened and the nurse started to walk back in before being stopped and pulled back by the doctor to give us some space.

A social worker would be in soon to chat and help us process the news. My mind raced while we waited for her to arrive, and I asked Brian to look up the survival rates for kidney cancer. He pulled up a search on his phone and stared silently at it for a while. I wasn't sure I wanted to find out what those rates were, but I also knew there was no way I was getting through the night without knowing. "It sounds like stage one is often cured with surgery, a survival rate of ninety-three percent."

Wow, okay, those sounded like good odds, but what did stage one mean? Time to Google the definition.

Stage 1: The cancer has not spread, is only in the kidney, and isn't larger than 7 centimeters.

Hmm, okay, the doctor had mentioned the tumor on my kidney was twelve centimeters and that it had spread to my liver, so that disqualified me from that. What was the next stage?

Stage 2: The cancer has not spread and is only in the kidney but is larger than 7 centimeters.

Since mine was twelve centimeters, it seemed like it could fit in that category if those spots in my liver weren't actually tumors. What were the survival rates for that?

The next stat was for regional spread, which the article described as the cancer spreading from outside the kidney to nearby structures or lymph nodes. It didn't say anything about stage two, but from the description, we wondered if nearby structures could mean the liver. Neither of us was medically trained; it felt like we needed a definition for these definitions. Brian read off the survival rate for regional spread: 71 percent. Still not great, but not terrible. I could be part of that 71 percent. Not knowing if I fell into this category or not, he continued.

Stage 3: The cancer may be any size, but it has spread to nearby sites outside of the kidney.

This sounded a bit more like it matched the regional description. So maybe I was stage three? We were still thoroughly confused by what "nearby" meant, so I asked what the final stage was.

Stage 4: The cancer has spread away from the kidney to distant sites or organs. The most common locations

*kidney cancer spreads or metastasizes to include dis-
tant lymph nodes, the lungs, bones, liver, and brain.*

We had our answer. The liver was considered a distant
organ. My stomach sank. Could I really be stage four? Afraid
of the answer, I asked what the odds were for stage four. In a
soft, defeated tone, Brian replied, "Eight percent."*

My eyes welled up with tears. Crushed, I muttered out a
response. "That's not zero . . ." I looked down toward my feet
at the end of the bed and repeated softly back to myself, "Eight
percent isn't zero . . ." I looked back over at Brain, tears pouring down my face. "I'm going to beat this . . . I'm going to fight;
eight percent isn't zero. It's not impossible. Even if there's only
a one percent chance I can make it, I can beat it," I insisted.

His tears matched mine as they fell from his eyes, trailing
into his beard. "Yes you will."

I didn't believe a word coming out of my mouth. Who was
I to think I would be the one to defeat the odds? Just an hour
earlier, I couldn't even get through a CT scan without a panic
attack. Surely, the victors over cancer were much stronger than
I. But the words provided a comforting distraction that we'd
repeat through the onslaught of tears, trying to convince ourselves this wasn't the end.

Within a few minutes, the door opened again. This time,
a woman walked in with a clipboard and introduced herself as
Lisa, the social worker on staff for the evening. She pulled up a
chair and said, "Tell me what's going on."

---

* Thanks to advancements in treatments, that number has since risen.

— 4 —

They said I was too young for cancer.

"THEY THINK IT'S cancer," I shared as emotion filled my voice and the disbelief creeped back in. "But they said I was too young for cancer," I whispered as the tears gave way.

"Who said you're too young for cancer?" Lisa replied in a soft and concerned tone. I struggled to speak through the tears, but after a few deep breaths, in an attempt to regain my composure, I tearfully walked Lisa through my history and how we'd ended up here.

It all began about a year and a half before I landed in the ER, when my blood pressure was flagged for the first time.

I'd recently moved to Utah after my grandmother passed and had set up an appointment with a new ob-gyn for an annual check-up. As they were grabbing vitals, I watched the shock on the nurse's face after she caught the reading. "One sixty-five over one sixteen. That can't be right." The cuff reinflated as she ran it again. "One sixty-three over one fifteen . . . do you normally have high blood pressure?" she asked, confused.

I didn't think I'd ever had an issue with it before, but honestly, I'd never really checked, and it'd been years since I'd been to a doctor. I remembered feeling winded as I walked up the stairs of the building to get to the office. Not knowing how blood pressure worked or even understanding how high those numbers were, I'd told her I'd been quite tired and just finished an energy drink before walking in. "Maybe that's why it was high?" I suggested.

"Maybe," she said as she nodded her head, logged the reading into the chart, and let me know the doctor would be in soon.

A blood pressure that high in a twenty-eight-year-old should have been a red flag, but I had no idea just how high it was, and the doctor never brought it up, so I didn't think much of it. Instead, in the appointment, we focused on getting me up-to-date with my Pap smear, and I asked about the new painful cramps I'd been getting.

I didn't think they were menstrual cramps, as they never coincided with my period—normally, they were at their worst a week beforehand—but they were extremely painful and would double me over anytime they appeared. The doctor assured me it was pretty normal and could still be menstrual cramps, as some women get cramps the week before their period begins. They didn't feel normal; the cramps were debilitating at times, and I'd never experienced them with that degree of pain. I began to wonder if I'd developed a low pain tolerance over the years and just needed to suck it up. Feeling embarrassed, I dropped it, and we wrapped up the appointment.

That summer, I continued to struggle with the cramps but had slowly learned the cycle and triggers at which they seemed to appear. They were always at their worst about a week before my period, and especially when I ate specific foods. So I started avoiding anything that would trigger the pain. I didn't eat before going out to ensure they never hit me at inconvenient times and pretty much accepted this was my new normal. Over the next few months, I also battled with extreme fatigue and mood swings that would hit me out of nowhere. I chalked it up to the fact that I'd just gone through a few major life changes, my grandma had passed, and I was in the middle of trying to switch careers.

But just a few months later, I reached a breaking point. I'd gone back to work full-time, this time in a new role as a software engineer, and I had just been given my first project to work on. I'd been struggling with the code but wanted to prove myself, so I was working fourteen-hour days, determined to figure it out. But by the end of the week, I was running on very little sleep and had a splitting headache that I couldn't shake. I also had some nausea setting in and had become lightheaded when I walked around. I started Googling for headache relief and causes before coming across high blood pressure as a common culprit in several of the results. I remembered how the nurse at my ob-gyn appointment seemed shocked by my blood pressure. I wondered if it still might be high. Since Advil and Tylenol weren't working, I bought a blood pressure monitor to check if that could be the cause.

When I got home, I opened the package, sat down, followed the instructions, and tried to match my positioning to the picture. I pressed start, and it began to inflate around my wrist, squeezing tighter and tighter. When I saw 157/110, I looked at the chart on the instruction manual. My reading was clearly into the red zone. *Could that explain my headache?*

The anxiety continued to build as I turned to my trusty friend Google again to find out how high blood pressure can be before you need to be concerned, but I found mixed and conflicting answers. I decided to call my mom, whose best friend was a physician assistant, to ask her if I should be worried as I continued to retest. 162/115, 163/117 . . . the readings were consistent but slightly rose as my anxiety built. With consistent readings over 160/115 paired with not feeling well, my mom suggested I get it checked out either by a doctor or the urgent care. I didn't have a primary care physician at the time. Being young, in my twenties, I hadn't ever seen the need. Hindsight's 20/20. After this event kicked off my health journey, I'd find myself with several PCPs along the way, trying to find the right fit and in pursuit of answers to my symptoms.

After grabbing one final reading at 170/120, I decided to heed the advice. As the urgent care did their workup, they clocked my resting heart rate at 165 and sent me straight to the ER for the rapid heart rate. After a whole lot of waiting, a couple labs, and an EKG that showed a fast but otherwise normal rhythm, they kept me for a few hours until my blood pressure dipped below 140/110, told me it was likely just anxiety, then sent me home with a pamphlet on panic attacks. They recommended I follow up with my primary care and a cardiologist to rule anything else out, which would soon kick off the wild-goose chase I'd find myself on for the next year.

For the rest of 2019 and all of 2020, I found myself in and out of nine different doctors' offices, looking for answers. Each one was surprised by my heart rate and confused by my high blood pressure at such a young age, but all of them came to the same conclusion again and again: it was anxiety. By the end of 2020, I'd had three different anxiety diagnoses added to my chart—generalized anxiety, social anxiety, health anxiety—a referral to a psychiatrist, and a workup for both OCD and PTSD.

I'd battled with anxiety most my life, and although I knew this was different, I couldn't find a way to properly communicate it. This wasn't just fleeting moments of anxiety from standing onstage or presenting to a roomful of people, the kind that subsides when you move out of the spotlight. This was a struggle I had every day. With a heart rate that often hovered around 135 to 160, it felt like I was constantly running a marathon while being chased by a bear. This was not normal.

However, I didn't have the language to communicate and convey that properly. I struggled to stand behind my convictions when challenged and didn't have confidence in speaking about my symptoms. When people share my story these days, the relentless advocating I had to do for myself often becomes a highlight. But the reality is that it was a skill born out of necessity, not nature, and I was absolutely miserable at it in the early days.

Every time I walked into an appointment, sat down, and it came time to talk about my symptoms, I'd start listing them off:

- Fatigue
- Loss of appetite
- Weight loss
- Diarrhea
- Hair thinning
- Abdominal cramps
- Rapid heart rate
- High blood pressure
- What felt like swollen lymph nodes in my neck
- High platelets
- Periodic night sweats

I'd only get about halfway through the list before I'd watch them glance at my chart and see their body language shift. I knew what that meant. They'd spotted the anxiety workup in my history and were now processing this information through a new filter. So when it came time for follow-up questions, fearing judgment, I'd always retreat.

The abdominal cramps that came around the same time every month, was I sure they weren't menstrual cramps? I didn't think so, but I guessed they could be.

Fatigue, loss of appetite, and hair thinning often present with stress. Had I been feeling anxious lately? It would have been lying to say no. Since we'd found my rapid heart rate and high blood pressure in the ER, I'd been living in a constant state of worry as I searched for answers.

Naïve to the medical system as well as a people pleaser, I took these questions as an evaluation of my character, not an opportunity to add clarifying detail. They were the experts. Who was I to disagree with their suggestions? The issue began to compound as I slowly began adopting their explanations as my own whenever I presented to a new provider or returned for follow-up.

Soon, I started focusing on the main symptoms that affected my day-to-day: the rapid heart rate and high blood pressure. These were areas that I was often far more worried about than the doctors I was seeing. They were convinced it was anxiety and that we needed to get it under control, but I was convinced it was a bigger issue. Which only, in turn, amplified the anxiety, resulting in a vicious circle. And I left the rest of my symptoms as honorable mentions as time permitted, typically followed by my own disclaimers and dismissals so I wouldn't sound like a hypochondriac with a long laundry list of issues.

My hair thinning and abdominal cramps became add-ins I'd toss in at the end as they were wrapping up and asking if there was "anything else." The way I described them evolved over time as well. The debilitating abdominal pain that at times would buckle me over and take my breath away until it passed . . . that became cramps that didn't line up with my period and were a bit more painful but weren't persistent, so "I don't know if I should worry about it." I was indeed quite worried about it, and secretly I hoped they would be too, so we could fit it into the workup. But I was too worried that if it panned out to be nothing, I'd just come across as weak or dramatic. I was already struggling to be heard. I didn't need to give them another reason to tune me out.

I continued to pursue the rapid heart rate and high blood pressure. Over time, as I became more comfortable following up and pushing for tests, they began ruling things out one by one, but as each result came back negative, I started to feel discouraged.

Through a cardiology workup, I received a heart rate monitor, stress test, and echocardiogram. When they all came back normal, my cardiologist added yet another tally to the anxiety diagnosis. I tried to share with him that I felt like something was wrong, like my body was having to work harder to pump the blood around. Not being medically trained, I couldn't think of another description. In search of answers and embarrassed, I even asked if it could be cancer. The cardiologist sounded slightly annoyed by the question and informed me that that wasn't for him to determine, but no, I was far too young for cancer. He recommended I follow up with my PCP, who could get me on something to help take care of the excessive worry, which he thought might improve my symptoms. In the meantime, he started me on a medication to try to lower my heart rate.

That wouldn't be the first or the last time I'd hear the phrase "You're too young for cancer." It'd find its way into several more conversations with other providers, typically in the exact same fashion, with a suggestion that I get on an antidepressant to get my anxiety under control.

One of the comments came in response to my asking for a scan to see if we could rule out cancer when I was frustrated that the medications weren't working. The doctor advised me not to go looking for problems, that I was too young for cancer, and that if we were to scan me, we'd be exposing me to unnecessary radiation. "Plus, once you go looking, you can't turn back the clock," they said. "Just about everyone will find something if you look hard enough, and when you pull something out of that box, you can't put it back in." They insisted that I was young and healthy and I should really focus on enjoying my life instead.

While these interactions sound problematic in the context of my situation, I am not sure many others would have handled me differently. I was frustrated by the lack of answers and what felt like an inability to get anyone to truly listen, but this wasn't a problem with any one doctor. It wasn't a physician problem, this was a system problem. I saw many different providers between April 2019 and December 2020. During this period, I met with three PCPs, a cardiologist, a cardiac electrophysiologist, an ENT, and three ob-gyns, and for the most part, they were all variations of the same appointment. We'd

talk about my concerns, they'd suggest I start an antidepressant for my anxiety, and I'd tell them I'd think about it but
would ask if we could order x test to rule out y, just for peace of
mind. As long as it wasn't a CT scan, they usually did. I believe
the majority of them genuinely wanted to help. No one wants
to let a twenty-eight-year-old walk out of their office with stage
four cancer. They saw sitting before them an extremely anxious young woman, refusing antidepressants, who wouldn't let
go of the idea that something else was wrong when test after
test came back normal. Anxiety was the easy conclusion for
them to jump to. In my opinion, they didn't have the time or
the systems to support them in doing a thorough workup.

Over time, and the more I've learned about both the medical system and our health in general, the more I've come to
understand the decisions each of them made, and I don't hold
resentment or animosity. Even comments like "Don't go looking for problems," while phrased and explained poorly at the
time, are actually rooted in logic. If you were to randomly scan
a hundred healthy individuals, you would likely come back
with several incidental findings—many of which were either
benign, wouldn't cause anyone any harm within their lifetime, or were transient and would have resolved on their own
by the next scan. However, when you find these things, you
have to follow up. You have to order the biopsy, you have to do
the surgery, or remain on a follow-up schedule until the issue
resolves. All of which comes with its own risks, complications,
financial toxicity, and A lot of emotional distress for patients
as they undergo diagnostics, some of which can be serious or
life-threatening.

While there are definitely gaps in the system and there are
things both my doctors and I could have done differently to
identify the issue sooner, I now understand how we ended up
here. But those learnings and understandings certainly took
time to develop, and as a relatively naive twenty-nine-year-old
who'd just had a stage four cancer diagnosis dropped into her

lap, I could see no logic or reason the night I received the news. All that came to me were the haunting words I'd heard again and again: "You're too young for cancer."

Back in the ER, I walked Lisa through a shortened, high-lighted version of the last year and a half. The appointments, the tests, the reassurance time after time that my symptoms were nothing more than anxiety. Devastated, defeated, and disappointed, through a wave of tears, I told her, "I feel like I slipped through the cracks." As I traversed the memories of every doctor's office I'd sat in and every missed opportunity to catch it, I was bitter and hurt. *Why didn't anyone listen?* My story seemed to weigh heavy on Lisa as she apologized that this had happened to me. I could tell she was just as disap-pointed with the system as I was.

Before we were discharged for the evening, I ended up ask-ing Dr. Morgan if anyone with stage four cancer ever makes it. I again felt the weight of the words in his response. He clari-fied his lack of knowledge about kidney cancer specifically but commented on the advancements they'd made in treatments over the past few decades and on how, in general, there were some people with late-stage cancers who had seen remissions. I could sense the tension between not wanting to set unreal-istic expectations and still wanting to provide us with a sense of hope. I thanked him and told him I didn't need to know the specifics, I just needed to know it was possible. "I'm going to fight it; I can beat it," I declared.

Lisa, who'd shared her battle and victory with a serious illness with me in our talks earlier, chimed in from the cor-ner of the room, "Yes, you will, and when you do, make sure you come back and say hi; we'll celebrate together." I promised both of them I would.

— 5 —

I struggle knowing all the dreams this house represents for me. It was our future, it's the family we planned to raise in it and all the memories and traditions I couldn't wait to start. It feels irresponsible to visit now. Like I'm visiting someone else's home.
                                        —Instagram post, January 23, 2021

IT WAS SEVEN AM on New Year's Eve by the time Brian and I left the hospital—eight hours after we'd arrived. We were exhausted and at a complete loss as to what would come next. I was surprised that they'd discharged me. I didn't know anything about cancer at the time, but the handful of people I'd heard who'd been diagnosed with cancer had been admitted and started chemo immediately. I certainly didn't want to be in the hospital, but I was worried being out meant I'd fall between the cracks again. Would they just forget about me over the holidays?

Sleep-deprived and with bloodshot eyes, Brian and I arrived home in a zombielike state. I went straight upstairs to Baxter, my little ten-pound Yorkie mix, who'd become my security blanket after years of adventures and heartbreak together. I cried as he excitedly spun in circles at my feet, welcoming me home. This tiny fur ball of energy had no idea what had just transpired, nor would he ever. Tail wagging, he was just excited we were home.

I wished I could forget what had just happened, but I couldn't stop the intrusive thoughts that accompanied me as I grabbed his leash and took him outside. I'd gotten Baxter as a puppy seven years prior amid a failing marriage. I'd always wanted a dog, but my ex-husband at the time wasn't much of an animal or dog person. I'd accepted that animals would never be a part of our lives. So I was surprised when he'd found Baxter through a Craigslist ad one day and asked if I wanted to go see him.

We weren't even a year into our marriage, but things were already on the rocks, which wasn't too surprising, given our relationship's on-again, off-again nature over the four years prior. With our relationship's fragility, getting a dog seemed less than ideal, but the answer to whether I wanted a puppy was always going to be yes. Have you ever heard of people who have a baby trying to fix their marriage? Yeah, that was us, but with a little four-pound fluffy tan puppy instead. Spoiler alert: it didn't exactly work.

Since then, Baxter and I had been through a divorce, new relationships, moves, road trips, and a whole lot of heartbreak together. He was my rock and my one constant. I had wondered at times what I'd ever do without him, a thought that would often bring me to tears, and I'd try to convince myself I'd never have to; he was going to live forever. Except now, as I watched his tiny paws prance around, avoiding the cold cement, I looked at him for the first time and wondered what he would do without me. The tears made the bite of a bitter-cold morning even more miserable as I hurried back inside.

What exactly is one supposed to do when you arrive home with this kind of news? Was I supposed to start a bucket list, quit my job, plan grand vacations, or prepare my will? I'd never been close with someone who'd been diagnosed with stage four cancer before, so my only point of reference was quite honestly from movies. You know, the ones where the patient is diagnosed with terminal cancer, then spends the rest of their days traveling the world, falling in love, and doing all of their favorite things before their disease catches up with them.

That sounded exhausting. Instead, Brian and I settled for crawling back into bed and watching movies on repeat, only breaking to refuel on snacks. We tried to get some sleep, but both of us were up most of the day. I told Brian I'd try to stay off Google, something I only succeeded at until I found myself lying there with my phone and my racing thoughts as he caught up on sleep. Every few minutes, I came across something that sent me down another spiral, but I just couldn't stop. I was hoping just one more search, one more click would lead to answers spelling out my future with any degree of certainty. Instead, I found a bunch of depressing stats and vague answers.

As night came, I watched with envy as friends rang in the new year and set their resolutions. The year 2020 had been a doozy for us all; merely making it through was a reason to celebrate. But the only thing that felt worth celebrating at the moment was the tiny sliver of vision I had left through my tear-swollen eyes to watch everyone's highlights online. Living vicariously through their celebrations. I'd be lying if I said I wasn't jealous; that was supposed to be us. In a matter of twenty-four hours, my list of New Year's resolutions had gone from buying a house, having a baby, and taking a honeymoon to simply not dying. It hardly seemed fair in the final year of my twenties, but I guess it beat the alternative.

When Brian and I first got together, I was still convinced Utah was only a temporary return for me and that, ultimately, I'd find my way back to Austin. I might have been born in Utah, but I'd spent most of my adult life in Austin, and after traveling the country and visiting other cities, I'd always been drawn back to it. As my lease was ending in the first few months Brian and I were dating, it felt too early to move in together, but I couldn't bring myself to sign another lease and commit to Utah. So I'd flown back to Austin in search of clarity and an apartment.

The second I landed, everything felt like home. It was the humidity and the smell of rain in the air, the beauty of the lights that lit up the skyline downtown, and the familiarity of a city that had shaped me into the person I'd become. This was home; the only thing it was missing was Brian. As I returned after a wonderful trip and visit with friends, I knew I had a difficult decision on my hands. Brian had recently started a new job and at the time was unable to move. But I had been too jaded by previous relationships to have faith that things would work out if I stayed. So after much deliberation, I made the decision to return to Austin, and through a mess of tears and smeared makeup, Brian and I called it quits.

That breakup lasted all of twenty-four hours before we both regretted the decision and knew we couldn't live without each other. Instead, Brian offered for me to move in with him in his tiny little condo for a few months while we gave our relationship a fair shot. If we broke up, I wouldn't be stuck in a lease, and I could go back to Austin. If we didn't, we'd stay in Utah together for a few years, then decide together where our forever home would be.

I moved from my small, temporary, and unfurnished apartment into Brian's condo, which was furnished with a mixture of his possessions and the secondhand furniture left behind. Since I worked remotely, we set up my desk and a space for me in the living room, which also served as Brian's office and a gaming room. Walking into the space, straight through the front door you'd find a room rich with nostalgia—a large textured floor lamp straight out of the nineties, an assortment of hand-me-down furniture, and an array of cat perches that'd been collected over the years. While my place didn't have enough furniture, his had a bit too much, and we had to get creative merging our lives to fit everything in. We were thrilled to be living together but knew this place wouldn't provide a long-term space for us to grow in. So, after a few months as our relationship progressed, we found a larger place to call home.

The townhome we settled on had only two rooms but more than double the square footage, with a large kitchen, high ceilings, and even a two-car garage—a true luxury after months of street parking in the snow. It was the perfect place to springboard our relationship and start building our lives together. And that square footage sure came in handy once COVID hit.

We enjoyed the townhouse and our time there, but when we got engaged, we began focusing on the next chapter of our lives. At first, we started looking for smaller homes, since we didn't plan on being in Utah long term. However, prices were climbing, everyone was in bidding wars, and any home that started within our budget quickly escalated beyond it. We began looking at building instead to lock our price in without risking a bidding war. However, these houses weren't starter homes and were at the top of our budget, so if we decided to build, we needed to talk about putting down roots.

I was pretty hesitant about putting down roots in Utah, but with two more years before Brian's job would give him flexibility to move, marriage on the horizon, and plans for kids, I knew Utah was the most logical choice. So we came to a compromise. I could get on board with staying, but only for our forever home. I was done moving. If we were planting these roots, we were planting them, and this would be where we raised our family.

After a couple months of looking, Brian and I found the perfect house, in the perfect neighborhood, with a perfect view overlooking the snowcapped mountains through the oversized windows in the living room. We picked out every detail together, from the floor plan and paint colors to finishes and the number of outlets in each room, building our white-picket-fence dream home that we planned to grow old in together.

But now, on top of the heavy weight of the diagnosis, I was worried about what Brian and I would do about our new home. It was our first big purchase together, and it had become far more than just a house for us. It was the representation of the future we were building. Although we hadn't decided to give it up yet, the very thought of doing so was enough to bring me to tears. It no longer felt like our dream but the representation of either Brian alone in an empty house that was supposed to house our future or the birthplace of another family's memories, the ones we'd never have a chance to make.

Brian hadn't asked to marry the girl with cancer, but here we were, and every ounce of love I had for him was now also filled with the pain I knew I would cause him one day when I passed. Having to come to terms with your own mortality is difficult enough, but the pain from imagining my loved ones carrying on without me was truly gut-wrenching and enough to bring me to my knees. I was determined to keep trying, but it was difficult to stay positive when even my happiest memories were accompanied by so much pain.

I spent the week between the ER trip and my first appointment consumed by a combination of fear, depression, and copious amounts of tears. I continued to doomscroll, looking through various cancer organizations and hospital websites. I became increasingly distressed as I found conflicting answers that, at the time, I didn't understand how to translate or sort through. Everyone kept telling me to be strong and stay positive, but what exactly did being "strong" mean? If you told me I was going to need strength to run a marathon, I'd spend the next few months training, preparing, and slowly building up my endurance. But for this, there was no guide. How could I build strength if I didn't even know what I was training for?

As a software developer, I was used to scouring the internet, looking for answers to problems. But the difference between a good search and a bad one is the base knowledge and context you take into it to filter through the results.

Which is exactly what I was missing as I searched for answers in the days leading up to my first appointment. I knew absolutely nothing about cancer, which was a recipe for disaster as I searched for answers on my prognosis without context to interpret the results.

This daily compulsion became so bad that I even asked Brian to check in on me anytime I was on my phone too long to keep me from looking anything else up and from spiraling myself into a depression, which worked pretty well until it didn't. I'd later find a small source of solace in discovering how common it is among patients to doomscroll. A group of dear friends who I met in the weeks that followed, endearingly referred to as the Chromophobe 6, would informally develop a pact around it: "Friends don't let friends doomscroll alone." First rule of doomscrolling: don't. Second rule of doom scrolling: if you break rule number one, no doomscrolling alone.

I'd do well when I was with Brian or when I could drown out negative thoughts with endless hours of Netflix. But the second I was alone, all the thoughts would creep right back in. Brian was my rock, and I leaned heavily on him to get through each day, but I found myself shielding even him from some of my most painful thoughts and questions during this time. After all, this was happening to both of us, and as much as he put on a strong front for me, he was going through his own grief. The last thing I wanted was to cause him more pain.

I kept finding myself drawing hot baths, hoping to relax, then ruining it by spending the entire time on my phone, digging for answers, each time sending myself into a deeper and deeper spiral. One night, I pushed it a little too far.

As I got into the tub after successfully staying off my phone the majority of the day, I made a rule to limit myself. I'd have ten minutes, then I had to put down the phone and actually relax. However, that night, one thing led to another, and before I knew it, two hours had passed, all the water had drained from the tub, and I was curled up, trying to catch my breath as the tears uncontrollably poured out from my eyes. What had started with a simple search had turned into a deep dive on the prognosis of liver metastases and a misinterpretation of more papers than I could count, ending in me coming to the conclusion that I likely only had eighteen months, at best, to live.

As one could imagine, I wasn't handling it well.

All I could think about was what that eighteen months might look like. Brian and I were supposed to be enjoying the first year of our marriage, but instead, he'd likely be caring for me as I slowly began to fall apart. We'd signed up for sickness and health, but sickness wasn't supposed to come this soon. Thirty was too young to watch your new bride slowly wither away in front of your eyes.

I then thought of my parents, who'd be forced to bury their own child. My siblings who'd be losing a sister; nieces and nephews, an aunt, and my best friend of over twenty years losing a confidant, a shoulder to lean on, and a lifetime of friendship. Imagining the pain I'd feel losing any of them, I absorbed the unimaginable grief. It felt like a dagger piercing through my chest. I continued to spiral, the tears splashing down and the despair echoing off the bathroom walls until the weight became too much to bear. I started to question if it was better for me to go now instead of dragging out the pain I'd slowly inflict on everyone around me and began contemplating how to do it. My searches became heavier as I switched from survival stats to states with Death With Dignity laws, overdosing, and the quickest ways to take my own life.

My spiraling thoughts were abruptly interrupted with a knock on the door. It was Brian, who'd noticed I'd been gone for a while and had come upstairs to check on me. "You okay in there?" he gently asked through the door, clearly hearing my tears on the other side. We sat in silence as I contemplated my options. I could tell him I was fine, something that neither of us would believe but that I knew would result in him giving me the space I needed to process through the emotions, or I could admit I was on the brink of disaster.

Typically in moments like this, I'd isolate myself from the world until I could pull myself through the other side. I'd walk through fire for anyone else, but I struggled with the idea of others shouldering my pain. It'd often amplify the emotions of what I already felt and add worry that I'd become a burden to anyone who'd outstretched their hand. But this time was different; I knew I was digging this hole too deep to get out on my own. With my head in my hands, staring at the bottom of an empty tub with tears rolling down my face, I whispered quietly, "I'm not."

Sensing the resignation in my voice, he asked if he could come in. I declined his request, not wanting him to see me this way. So he sat on the corner of the bed a few feet away and began talking to me through the door instead. Trying to piece things together without pushing, he gently asked what had happened and if I had been on my phone. Both defeated and ashamed, I admitted I had, then paused briefly as I choked back the tears. "It's not good . . ."

"What's not good?" he asked. I felt his patient restraint as he sat tight on the edge of the bed when I knew all he wanted was to be by my side.

"All of it." I erupted into tears again as I struggled to get out the rest. "The prognosis with liver metastasis . . . it's not good," I said as the emotion rushed over me and I began hyperventilating. "I don't know if I'll even have a year."

I heard the concern in his voice as he tried to calm me down. "Just breathe; it's okay. Just breathe with me . . ." He offered a big inhale that I tried to match.

I took a deep breath, then another, and another, slowly calming until a thought reentered and retriggered the cycle once again. I closed my eyes and continued to focus on my breathing. *One breath in. One breath out.* I tried to block out all other thoughts. Breath by breath, I came back down, and the tears slowed.

Brian and I sat silently for a while, breathing together on opposite sides of the door until he asked me to come out and sit with him. I agreed this time, pulled myself out of the tub, threw back on the sweats I'd been living in for the past three days, and opened the door.

The second I saw him, I was reminded of how lucky I was to have him in my life, and the tears came rushing back. He reached for my hand and guided me to the bed, where I collapsed into his embrace. "I don't want to lose you." I buried my tear-soaked face into his chest.

"You never will," he reassured me as he pulled me close. We sat wrapped in each other's arms until I finally verbalized the feeling for the first time. "I'm scared," I said, my head still pressed against his chest. "I'm not ready to die."

He squeezed me tightly, his whole body wrapping me in a strong embrace, before pulling back to look me in the eyes. "You're not going to," he assured me.

"But I am; it's only a matter of time . . ." I battled the emotion as I felt the weight of the words falling from my mouth. "I'm scared, and I know it's only going to get worse." The guilt was mounting. As difficult as this moment was, I knew this was only the beginning. This likely wouldn't be the last time Brian would have to pick me up off the floor.

He took my hands. "I'm scared too, but we're going to get through this together," he declared with unwavering commitment.

I didn't deserve him. He didn't deserve this. I imagined the heartache I'd bring one day if and when I didn't "get through this." The pain was all-consuming. "I don't want to do this to you. You don't deserve this." I collapsed back into him. The only thing that felt worse than dying itself was the idea of leaving him behind. I didn't know how either of us would make it through this.

Searching for a solution, I asked, my voice cracking, "Would it be better for me to go now, so I don't put us both through the pain?"

His eyes instantly welled up with tears. "What, no, what are you talking about?" he desperately pleaded.

As the tears streamed down my face, I repeated myself. "Would it be easier for me to end it, so I don't cause any more pain? If it'll be easier to let go of me now, I can, I can go now . . ." I was sobbing uncontrollably and couldn't believe the words coming out of my mouth. I was willing to do anything to lessen the pain I knew my passing would bring to those I loved most, even take my own life. This wasn't like me.

I watched my words crash into Brian like a ton of bricks. He lost his composure and began crying uncontrollably alongside me. "Absolutely not. No, Katie, please. I don't care what it looks like; I don't care how hard it is. I want to spend every last second I have left with you. Please don't take that away from me," he pleaded as his arms fully consumed me in an embrace once more, and I felt his tears slip onto my shoulder. "Promise me."

My intention was never to hurt him; I wanted to cause him less pain, not more. I tightly squeezed him back. "I promise I won't . . ."

We both held the embrace and refused to let go. I don't think either of us could believe I'd let the words come out and that I'd just spoken them with such honest intent. This wasn't who I was. It was clear I was slipping fast. I needed help.

I'd been struggling with debilitating amounts of fear and anxiety since leaving the ER and already had an appointment set at Huntsman to meet with a psychiatrist. But that appointment wasn't for another week. So in an effort to find help and hoping to find others who might also have a kidney cancer diagnosis that I could relate to, I began browsing Instagram hashtags, looking for hope.

Most of the patient-directed content I found from cancer centers or hospitals felt like it wasn't geared toward patients my age. Which seems like a subtle detail, but it only added to the feelings of isolation. I couldn't relate to the sixty-five-year-old man sitting across from his doctor or the inspirational photo of a woman surrounded by her grandkids still enjoying life's most meaningful moments. But on Instagram, I found patients my age or at least within a decade or two, and one in particular kept coming across my feed: Daniel.

He appeared to be in his early forties, well dressed, with twenty different pairs of bold circular glasses and a well-groomed salt-and-pepper beard. He had what he described as terminal stage four kidney cancer that he talked candidly about, but his page was filled with posts of him carrying on with life regardless. In one picture, he'd be getting an infusion or going for a CT scan, and in the next he'd be riding his bike, snuggling his new puppy, or marrying the love of his life. I admired both the honesty and humor in his posts, where he'd share his struggle to overcome side effects from treatment while also poking fun at the explosive diarrhea that earned him a trip to the hospital. Were we allowed to laugh at cancer? Still quite distraught over my own diagnosis, I wasn't sure how one ever reached that state of mind, but something about his posts felt relatable. This was my first glimpse into what life with cancer might be like, and while it certainly didn't sound glamorous, it sounded doable. Unsure if I'd get a response, I decided to send him a message.

Hey there, I'm not sure if you read messages from complete strangers but I was just diagnosed with kidney cancer w/metastasis to my liver on Wed. I'm 29 and terrified. Was wondering if I could ask you some questions and if you could share with me some of your story. Is it true that it's incurable once it's metastasized?

He replied the next morning: Hey Katie. Fancy a chat? Are you in the UK?

Fancy a chat? That had to be the most approachable way to start a conversation about cancer. I liked this guy already. The next thing he asked was how I was doing; he knew I was scared but wanted to know how I was feeling.

I said that physically I felt fine, maybe a little nauseous, but that I thought it was from all the emotion and that I was doing okay as of a couple days ago. I had accepted the diagnosis and was determined to fight, but that was all before I actually started researching what that meant for the type of cancer we had. I always figured I had options, chemotherapy, radiation or other options to fight it. Last night I took a tailspin learning kidney cancer doesn't respond to those treatments and I feel utterly helpless, I confided.

He didn't respond for a few minutes, and it looked like he was offline. So I decided to shower and attempt to get ready for the day while I waited for his reply. I headed into the bathroom but left my phone on the bed with Brian, honoring a new rule I'd set the night before of no longer bringing it in with me.

Once I finished and returned, Brian handed me the phone and told me I should check it, since it had been buzzing the entire time. I'd told him I was looking for other patients, and he'd seen me browsing Instagram the night before, but he didn't know I'd reached out to anyone yet. As I opened up my phone to seven new voice messages, I caught him up to speed, and we listened together.

As I pressed play, Daniel introduced himself with a patient, calming voice and a British accent. He confirmed that our type of cancer didn't typically respond to traditional treatment like chemotherapy but then started describing the immunotherapies and TKIs they used instead. He personally was currently on immunotherapy, which he began explaining before he was cut off by the end of the recording.

Brian and I looked at each other with a bit of relief as I hit play on the next message, where Daniel was back, now cussing out and laughing at the length of the voice message that he knew he was going to exceed again as he carried on anyway. "But whatever you do, don't go on Google and self-diagnose yourself and your cancer; it will drive you absolutely insane. And all you'll find is old reports and old clinical trials that won't really tell you anything but will put you in a tailspin. So stay off Google." I felt Brian squeeze my hand. He'd told me the same thing a hundred times already, but hearing it from another patient felt different. It seemed like I wasn't the only one who'd walked myself into a panic attack over too much Googling.

"Also, no, you're not going to die—that's ridiculous, you need to get that out of your head first," he advised with a passion and tone that was reminiscent of telling your 110-pound friend that no, they indeed do not look fat in the dress. He went on to share, "The road might get a bit bumpy for you, as it does for all of us, but don't be scared, because you're surrounded by amazing people." I felt a tear drop from the corner of my eye and splash onto the screen as I looked up at Brian, who was also glossy-eyed. It'd felt like we were alone, lost out at sea for days, but Daniel had just tossed us a map. Who knew the words from a stranger halfway across the world could resonate so deeply?

Daniel and I messaged back and forth for the majority of the morning as he provided advice and insight about the road ahead. He shared his journey, the treatments he had been on, and the incredible community of people he'd met along the way. He also encouraged me to appreciate each day and, even though life might change, to never stop living. He might have an incurable cancer, but he himself was engaged to be married to the love of his life next month. They'd just bought a puppy and looked forward to a life well lived together regardless of how long it'd be.

As our conversation came to an end, I thanked him for his honesty and openness as he welcomed me into the new family and community of patients I'd find here. You're in a new family now, and we've (I) have your back, he assured as he connected me with a few support groups and gave a parting reminder to stay off the internet unless it was to chat with other patients.

As he walked me back from the ledge that day, I learned the true power and importance of connecting with other patients. I knew I'd never be able to properly repay him but hoped as I embarked on a path of my own that I might pay it forward and provide the same comfort to other patients one day. In the meantime, the two of us would stay connected, rooting each other on from across the sea.

After my positive conversation with Daniel, instead of actively trying to think of things unrelated to the cancer, which had only backfired on me so far, I tried to focus on reframing or finding even the smallest ounce of positivity or light from the night I was diagnosed. Were there any silver linings? I mean, the outcome was miserable, but I had come across a few incredible people along the way. The first to come to mind was the CT tech who'd calmed me down as I had a panic attack during my first scan. I was grateful he was the one working that night. Then there was the doctor who'd ordered the ultrasound. If he hadn't put that order in, I'd likely have walked out of the ER, and we still wouldn't have any answers. As I zoomed out one level further, I focused on why I'd even ended up in the ER in the first place: Casey, the nurse practitioner from the urgent care.

As I recalled our conversations from that evening, my gratitude grew. Not only was Casey the first person to really take me seriously, but he was also the reason we'd finally found what was wrong. The doctor in the ER had ordered the ultrasound that found the tumor, but Casey had been the one to sound the alarm. Had it not been for his thorough examination and his reassurance that night, there was no saying when we would have found this thing. I didn't know where my diagnosis would lead from here, but regardless, I felt like this man had saved my life. I wished there was a way I could thank him.

I wanted to write him a thank-you card but wondered if that might be a little weird. How would I even get it to him? But after lingering on the thought, I decided, who cares if it's a little weird? I'd spent the majority of my life holding back, but life was obviously far too short to censor who you are. I didn't know too many people who had ever been offended by a thank-you. And if he was, what did I care? Seems I may die soon anyway . . . at best, I make someone's day; at worst, someone I'll probably never interact with again might think I'm a little weird. That seemed like a gamble I was willing to take. Plus, it felt nice to focus on doing something nice for someone else instead of being caught up in my own misery for a bit.

I wrote and rewrote the same message on the card four times before I got it right. Misspellings on one, teardrops on another, but eventually, I had one worth sharing, and I stuffed it in an envelope ready to deliver.

He'd been working the evening shift when I'd gone in a few nights prior, and since I didn't know when he'd be working next, I decided to head in around the same time. On the drive over, Brian and I stopped for a box of cookies from one of our favorite cookie shops to go with the card. I mean, who doesn't like cookies?

Once we made it to the urgent care, the nerves set back in, and I felt my heart rate take off. *Actually, maybe this is weird . . . People don't do this . . . I probably shouldn't do this . . .* I contemplated turning around and heading back home before Brian reassuringly reminded me, "You're doing something nice. You're dropping off a box of cookies; no one is going to hate you for leaving cookies. Just go inside, everything will be fine." It was exactly what I needed. I grabbed the cookies and the card and headed inside.

The nerves continued as I walked through the doors and up to the counter. What was I supposed to say? I wanted to get Casey this card. I wanted to thank him, but I hadn't exactly thought through the logistics of how this was all going to go down. As I got to the counter, I apologized for the odd question but told the woman behind the desk that I'd seen a nurse practitioner the other night whose name was Casey, and I wondered if he was working so I could drop him off a card. She looked confused as she tried to place who I was talking about. "Casey? Do you know his last name?"

I didn't. We went in circles with descriptions back and forth until she disappeared into the back to ask the rest of the team. I felt my eyes starting to well up with tears. *Of course, the first nice thing I try to do is a complete failure.* Had I not remembered his name correctly? I could have sworn his name was Casey.

After a few minutes, she reappeared. It turned out Casey didn't work at their location—he had helped out for one night due to understaffing—and she wasn't sure exactly which location he worked at.

A tear fell from the corner of my eye as I told her that I'd seen him a few nights prior and he'd sent me to the ER after finding a mass that would end up being stage four cancer, and that I really just wanted to say thank-you. If it weren't for him, I said, I felt like we likely might never have found it. Taken aback and clearly moved by the story, she reached out her arms, gesturing for the card and cookies. She didn't know where Casey was, but she'd do her best to find him for me. I thanked her, slid the box across the counter, and headed back to the car.

I reached the car, defeated and in tears, as Brian tried to piece together what possibly could have gone wrong in there. I told him I'd left the cookies and card behind but didn't think they'd ever make it to Casey, since he didn't normally work at that location and none of the staff working that night had worked with him or knew who he was. Wiping a tear from my cheek, Brian reached across the center console and pulled me close, reassuring me that it was the right thing to do anyway. Hopefully, the card would make it to Casey soon. As he started the car and we headed home, I was left wondering if my days would ever stop ending in tears.

— 6 —

Google and the internet are scary places for cancer patients but I'm grateful for this platform and the kindness and support of a complete stranger a world away, who's helped me connect to a new family and network of support.
—Instagram post, January 4, 2021

*W*HY IS IT *so taboo to talk openly about cancer, and why is it only something we talk about in the past tense, only sharing when someone has either passed or beaten cancer? Surely there is a whole lot that happens in between.* As I lingered on that thought, I remembered Chelsee, a girl I'd gone to high school with, who'd been diagnosed with lymphoma and documented her treatment and stem cell transplant on Instagram in 2019. I remembered how much I felt I learned from her without having a diagnosis myself. I wondered why more people didn't do what she did. *Wouldn't it be easier to know how to show up for people we care about if we had a better idea of the road they face?*

I thought about how many other patients, just like me, had probably been looking for the kind of information Chelsee had shared but had had to navigate the path on their own. I knew from searching for clues of what I might be up against from others who had walked a similar path—and coming up empty time after time—that they were in short supply. I mostly came across memory posts detailing a difficult journey and a hard-fought battle as family and friends mourned and paid tribute to their loved ones who'd passed. So I decided I would share the good, the bad, and the ugly of wherever this path was about to take me—hoping that one day it could help someone else know what to expect and feel a little less alone.

So, the morning after I got diagnosed, I drafted up a post that I decided to share on Facebook and Instagram.

This is what day 1 of a new cancer diagnosis looks like.

Last night I went to the ER for a dull pain and some swelling in my upper right abdomen. I left 7 hours later with a large tumor on my kidney that has spread to my liver and a Renal Cell Carcinoma diagnosis (kidney cancer).

This photo represents the full range of emotions I've felt over the past 24 hours. It's raw, unfiltered and full of pain.

I'd be lying if I said I wasn't scared of what lies ahead of me but after years of trying to convince an endless number of doctors something was wrong and having them dismiss me with an anxiety pre-scription and a "you're too young for cancer", I finally have a path and diagnosis to follow. Certainly not one I'd ever want but it was the cards I was dealt and now we're going to learn to play them.

When the doctor came in to explain my diagnosis, I didn't instantly burst into tears as I'd expected. I had known something was wrong and off in my body for a long time and for once, I had someone sitting across from me with compassion and I knew from that moment on, I'd have a full team of doctors in my corner and we'd take this journey on together.

I was heartbroken but felt relief in finally having some answers and a path forward.

We don't know what that path forward looks like quite yet, it's likely a late stage due to the spread and we'll get more news and staging next week once I meet with my doctors. But trying to be hopeful.

I created this account to share my journey with you all and to build awareness. I will show the good and the bad and each day I plan to make one post documenting what I'm struggling with for the day and one for what I'm grateful for. My first gratitude post dedicated to my incredible husband.

So come along for this journey and let's help me kick cancer!

The post accompanied a photo of me with swollen eyes, no makeup, and a beanie to cover the hair I couldn't be bothered to put up.

It was a difficult post for me to share. Up until that point, my social media had been a highlight reel of my life—sharing the wins, the vacations, and life events but keeping anything too personal tucked back behind the curtains. But after sharing, I was met with overwhelming love and support from friends, family, and acquaintances who'd been watching from a distance. With so many reaching out asking how they could help, sending food, and encouraging messages, I felt guilty for not responding to each. I certainly tried, but I could only get through a few characters of thanking them and expressing how much their messages meant before I'd become a puddle of tears. I read every single one several times. I was going through the most difficult chapter of my life, but I'd never felt so loved.

In an effort to try to "stay positive," I committed to highlighting at least one positive each day as I documented my path forward. But I'd also allow myself to highlight one thing I was struggling with each day too, as long as it came before my positivity post—my small attempt to find silver linings through what seemed like often impossible circumstances. Staying positive was a lot easier said than done after just having the rug ripped out from under me. Positivity was the absolute furthest emotion from my mind, but as I was confronted by the relentless recommendation around every corner, I decided to lean in.

It was a struggle. Every positive thought I had was also accompanied by feelings of sadness. In my first "positivity" post, I highlighted my gratitude for Brian: that I was grateful to have him by my side and for how much he supported and loved me every day, that I was thankful he had come into my life. All things I wholeheartedly felt and meant, but writing the words didn't bring joy; they brought an immense amount of pain as my gratitude shifted toward guilt and I thought about all the unexpected change and heartache I'd just introduced into our lives.

But I kept trying. By the second day, I took to crowdsourcing names for my tumor in an attempt to make light of the situation and to make this massive tumor growing inside of me feel a bit less intimidating. Newman, from *Seinfeld*, quickly arose as a leading contender, and after recalling an episode where Jerry refers to Newman as "pure evil," I couldn't imagine a more fitting name. Newman would now be how we referred to this giant unwelcome guest taking up residence in my body. All I could think about was his eviction day, which felt like it couldn't come soon enough as I struggled each day to keep my mind from focusing on what felt like slow, impending doom.

In the days that followed leading up to my appointment, I did my best to stay off Google. Instead, I focused on finding support groups, where I found hundreds of folks living, surviving, and thriving with their disease. Inspired by the openness and sense of community I saw in comments, I decided to make a post of my own, introducing myself, the extent of my disease, and sharing my fears about my first appointment.

I was nervous to share so openly, but within minutes, comments began rolling in from patients across the country, welcoming me with open arms, providing encouragement, and offering tips and questions to ask at my appointment. This must have been the family my new friend Daniel was talking about. I didn't know who these wonderful strangers were, but I no longer felt so alone; these were my people.

The comment section slowly grew and became a wealth of knowledge of everything I'd need to know for my first appointment and the road ahead. There were several recommendations to bring someone with me or to take a notebook of questions to ensure I didn't forget anything. Still unsure if Brian would be able to come with me or not, I began taking notes and writing down questions in case I became too emotional during the appointment to remember them.

I pulled out a pen and paper and wrote in large font across the top of the page, *Questions for Dr. Swami.*

1. What is the stage and grade of my cancer?
2. What is the subtype of kidney cancer?
3. Where has it spread?
4. What treatments are available?
5. Which one are we going to start me on, and why do you think it is the best to start with?
6. Will I be having surgery? If so, will it be on just my kidney or my liver as well?
7. What is my prognosis?

In hindsight, it's crazy to look back on moments like these and wonder how different life might have played out if each piece hadn't aligned the way it did. My journey is full of tiny catalysts that led to where I am today, but these support groups and Daniel's and my conversation that led me to them were certainly some of the most foundational ones. It was by his recommendation that I had joined the patient communities that became my lifeline. The connections and friendships I'd go on to build from and through these groups, like the Chromophobe 6 and many others who became dear friends, would quite literally save my life one day, and it all started with a little kindness, connection, and a British accent.

By the time appointment day rolled around, I had a full sheet and a half of questions queued up for my oncologist. I was walking in with what felt like a mountain of unknowns but felt more prepared and hopeful that I'd be walking out with answers and a clear path forward.

— 7 —

I was lost in the system of over a year as this tumor has been growing inside me and today I struggled feeling as if I was lost in the system all over again.
—Instagram post, January 8, 2021

MY FIRST APPOINTMENT was on January 6, 2021, at eleven thirty AM, on what would end up being a memorable day not just for me but for most of the country after everything that would unfold at the Capitol. The night before, I didn't sleep a wink.

Visitor restrictions were still in effect at most centers, and I was worried Brian wouldn't be able to come with me. So our plan was to have him wait in the car, and I'd ask if I could record the appointment—a recommendation from a patient in one of the support groups—or we would see if I could put him on speaker while I talked with the doctor. Neither option sounded particularly appealing, but I knew facing my own mortality while sitting alone in a cold hospital room chair would leave me too emotional to retain anything on my own. So we'd have to make do.

Huntsman Cancer Institute is located next to and a part of the University of Utah, where I'd gone to college. The dorms I'd lived in were less than a mile away, and I'd passed the building on the shuttle to and from class a hundred times before, but I'd never taken the time to appreciate it until now. The beautiful and prominent building sat on top of the hillside, overlooking the Salt Lake Valley with large panoramic windows and a grand, inviting entrance. As we turned into the garage, my heart began to race as the nerves mounted, and I wondered how a building this beautiful could house so much pain.

Once we parked, I began gathering my things as Brian rattled off a checklist of what I needed to bring inside. Insurance card—check. Driver's license—check. Notebook and a pen—check. A fully charged phone—check. I placed everything together in my lap and looked at Brian. There was still one thing I was missing: him. How was I possibly going to do this on my own? A tear fell from the corner of my eye and down my cheek as Brian wiped it away. "You can do this. It's going to be okay, and I'll be right here the whole time. Text me as much as you need to." We embraced in a long hug, and he kissed my forehead as I reluctantly opened the door, got out of the car, and headed inside.

The entrance from the garage led into the lower level of the building, where there was a young man checking for and distributing masks as patients entered. Nearly a year into the pandemic, life still felt so strange. I remembered thinking about moments like this early into the spread of COVID in March 2020, back when we were still doing strange things like wiping down our groceries. I remembered thinking about all the women delivering babies in hospital rooms alone, loved ones separated from family members during life-threatening emergencies, and cancer patients facing treatment or difficult news without someone by their side. My stomach always sank at the thought, but I never imagined I'd be in that position myself one day.

The man at the door passed me a mask as he called the elevator for us. We had to take it one by one up to the main entrance for a more thorough screening. Once upstairs, we queued into the screening at the front, where we'd sanitize, confirm a lack of symptoms, and have our temperature checked. I followed the couple in front of me step by step as we made it through the line. The woman appeared to be my age, and as she confirmed her appointment, I wondered how they'd gotten the clearance for her husband to come along. I made a mental note to ask the front desk if they had an updated policy once I checked in. If I could figure out where that was, that is. The entrance opened to a large open foyer with a grand staircase leading to the second floor, and I began skimming for signage or directions of where to go next as I funneled through the line.

When it was my time to be screened, I answered no to the long list of questions about COVID exposures and symptoms and stepped in front of the iPad set to check my temperature as I made my way to the greeter to give my name. She began shuffling through the papers on her clipboard, looking once, then again before reconfirming my name. "You said Katie Coleman? Do you have an appointment today?" she asked as she thumbed through the list.

"I think so. I'm supposed to have my first appointment, but I don't know if I'm in the right place," I nervously responded as I glanced over my shoulder, noticing the line queueing up behind me.

She flipped through the list once more. "Could it be under any other name?"

"Oh, Moosman, Kathryn Moosman," I responded. I turned beet red while she returned to the list, a bit perplexed. *Moosman.* I hadn't had a chance to complete my name change since getting married. I'd filled out all the paperwork but was waiting for an appointment with the driver's license division and social security office. Both were booked out for several months due to the pandemic.

"Ah, there you are," she confirmed, highlighting my name. She wrapped a band around my right arm that resembled the one from the ER I'd received the week before. I was used to getting these types of wristbands at concerts, events, and racetracks. Receiving them now in hospitals and appointments, I was not a fan of this rebranding.

Too embarrassed to ask for directions after holding up the line, I continued into the foyer and again began searching for a check-in desk or anything to direct me where to go. I must not have been hiding my confusion well; a nurse tapped me on the shoulder and asked if I was lost as I stood in the center of the room, looking up toward the second floor. I told her I was here for my first appointment but didn't know where that was. She asked the type of cancer I had, then escorted me to the front desk on the second floor so I could get checked in and ask if Brian could come in to accompany me. I felt bad for detouring her from wherever she was headed to but appreciated the help and thanked her as we parted ways.

As I scanned the room, I noticed just how much younger I was than everyone. There were only a handful of patients in the lobby, maybe five to ten at most, but all of them appeared to be over sixty. Feeling a bit isolated, I decided to take a seat at the back of the room but within earshot of the door so I could hear them call my name.

There was a walkway between me and the rest of the room. I watched as patients passed by, looking for anyone remotely close to my age, without much success. The incidence rate of stage four kidney cancer between the ages of twenty and forty-nine is under one thousand cases a year in the United States.

Being the youngest in the room by many decades felt lonely until I sat with the thought a little longer. I couldn't believe I'd actually been hoping to see someone my age. Cancer is not the kind of thing you wish for anyone; the fewer faces I saw here, the better.

I shifted my focus back to my upcoming appointment and began running through all the questions I had prepared. I was avoiding my phone like the plague to keep myself off Google, so this felt like the next best option. I got through my list of questions, made stars next to the most important ones, and started to wonder when the nurse at the front desk would let me know about Brian. She'd stepped away ten or fifteen minutes ago, and I hadn't seen her return. I anxiously shifted in my chair as I worried I might not have an answer before it came time for my appointment.

I decided to wait a few more minutes before making my way back up to the front desk. The nurse still hadn't returned, so I waited, hoping they'd eventually see me. A couple more minutes passed before she appeared again at the window. I followed up on the request for Brian to come in, and she looked around her desk as if she were looking for something, "Oh yes, sorry—we got a little distracted. Since it's your first appointment, as long as he goes through the same screening you did, he can come inside. What's his name? I'll run it down to let them know he's okay to come in."

Got distracted? I didn't know why, but that stung a little. I understood this was just another Monday for them, but I was literally about to go back into a room to have someone tell me if I was dying or not. This felt important. But at least now I wouldn't have to stomach that conversation alone. She took down Brian's name on a Post-it, and I texted him to let him know to come inside as I sat back down.

A few minutes passed, and I heard one of the nurses call my name to bring me back for labs. I gathered my things and followed her into an open room with large chairs lining the walls. My heart raced as I took a seat and wondered how the woman next to me appeared so calm, making small talk with the nurse while she poked and prodded her arms. I, on the other hand, was already apologizing to my nurse as I turned away and closed my eyes before she'd even found a vein.

I was terrified of needles, something I found to be a bit ironic now that I had cancer. But, I guess, the cancer couldn't get me if the needle took me out first! I'd been known to become lightheaded before having blood drawn, so I asked the nurse not to warn me as she went for the stick. The anticipation was always the worst part. She agreed, and as she began prepping the area, she made small talk instead. I appreciated the gesture. I could tell she was trying to distract me so I wouldn't see it coming, but unfortunately, it only made me that much more anxious.

Whenever I find myself in high-stress moments, what I need more than anything is silence as I talk myself through it. *You've got this. It's just a little stick; you barely even felt it last time. It's going to be over before you know it. Just breathe . . .* The pep talk from my inner dialogue loops over and over in my head, providing my own distraction and a self-soothing outlet to calm the panic. If I try to hold a conversation in these moments instead, my mind runs wild and I feel completely unprepared. Which is exactly where I found myself as I tried to answer questions about where I lived and what I did for a living as I felt a needle poke through my skin, catching me off guard. I stopped midsentence and took a few deep breaths to refocus. By the time I'd gotten through the second breath, I'd felt a quick pinch and felt the nurse begin applying pressure. "That's it, we're done. You did great!" she encouraged as she wrapped the site and sent me on my way.

It was never the pain from the needle that got to me but instead the anticipation itself. Which is a very fitting analogy for the entire diagnostic process with cancer—full of waiting and anticipation. A lot of sitting around, knowing something unpleasant is coming but not quite knowing when or how it will strike. So off I went back to the lobby, waiting for the rather unpleasant conversation I knew would be awaiting me soon.

As I came out, I saw Brian, who'd taken a seat in the same area I was sitting before, and I walked back to join him, relieved to have him there. We waited together for another hour until they called me back for my appointment. This was it, the moment I'd been both anxiously awaiting and dreading for the past week.

A physician assistant came in to greet us first, and we spent a solid thirty minutes recapping the events, symptoms, and doctors' appointments that had led us here, along with a full family history. I watched as the scribe meticulously took notes behind her. It felt surreal as I imagined what it must be like to be her in that moment, taking notes and detailing the slow spiral of a tearful, likely terminal cancer patient just a few years older than she was.

After we finished the preliminary questions, she paused to check in. The combination of having to relive the night I was diagnosed while openly discussing any risks or exposures for cancer was getting the best of me. I couldn't get through more than a few sentences before a new tear would trace its way down my cheek. She passed a box of tissues across the table as I took off my glasses to wipe the tears from my eyes, the heaviness of the conversation sinking in. "Don't worry, we're going to figure this out," she reassured me as she stood to make her exit, letting me know the doctor would be in shortly. She stepped out, and the door gently closed behind her.

Brian put his hand on my leg in a show of support, and I pulled several more tissues from the box. I turned and looked at him as I took off my mask, holding it from the strap between two fingers as it dangled below. "Little soggy . . . ," I said with a smirk, as if I hadn't just funneled a gallon of tears and snot into it. Self-deprecating humor, my go-to maneuver during stressful situations and my favorite coping mechanism.

He chuckled back, breaking the tension in the room. "I bet," he confirmed as we began bantering back and forth about our current predicament and I poked fun at how sexy his new bride was as I put my mask back on, fogging up my glasses. This was one of my favorite things about our relationship. I knew he'd always be there to support me through the toughest moments but was also there to laugh with me through them, which felt even more important at times.

As we laughed through the tears and the nerves returned, he squeezed my hand, which I knew was replacing the forehead kiss that'd typically follow this kind of anxious banter. A gentle gesture that was his way of saying, *You're ridiculous, but I absolutely love you for it, and everything's going to be okay.*

Before we knew it, the door opened again, and in walked Dr. Swami, who introduced himself before sliding over a stool to position himself across from us as he sat down. I opened my notes and saw the first item on the list with a big star next to it, reminding me to ask if we could record the appointment. I knew it'd be helpful for us to reference back to, so before we got started, I paused to ask. I was expecting him to say no, but he was quite supportive, providing an encouraging gesture and holding the conversation until we were ready. I'd replay this recording several times in the days that followed, and listening back to it now, it's like a portal to another lifetime.

As the conversation began, Dr. Swami let Brian and I know they'd reviewed and discussed my scans that morning at the tumor board, a meeting I'd later learn was a meeting held a couple of times a month, bringing together a multidisciplinary teams of doctors to review complex cases together. As a group, they'd identified two major problems. The first was the large mass growing on my kidney, and the second were spots they'd identified in my liver. I wasn't sure what a tumor board was at the time and was too busy trying to keep up with the conversation to ask.

He told us that the tumor on my kidney was quite large, and that when they came across tumors this size, they were often chromophobe kidney cancer (a rare type of kidney cancer), which often had been growing for many years. They might expect to see a tumor this size in someone in their late forties, fifties, or sixties, but it was a bit unusual in someone my age. They wanted to get a biopsy to take a better look and to check for any mutations.

Next, we discussed the plan for the lesions in my liver. Dr. Swami let us know that they couldn't be certain what the lesions were; it was possible they could be adenomas, which are benign growths that can grow in the liver. So he was going to send me for an MRI of my abdomen, which would provide us a better look to determine if we'd need to worry about or biopsy those lesions as well. Lastly, he wanted to send me for a brain MRI to rule out any spread, since I'd mentioned a few months prior I'd been seeing tiny specks in my vision, like when you stand up too quickly and feel lightheaded.

With a plan now in place, he paused for any questions. I glanced down at my notebook, scanning quickly for the ones I wanted to prioritize first. I'd had one burning question since the day we found it: how long had it been growing? He couldn't say with any certainty and mentioned they'd know more after the biopsy but said he suspected it had been growing for over a year.

When cancer spreads or grows quickly, it often presents with symptoms as it moves, pushes, and invades organs around it. However, when it grows more slowly, the body adjusts and accommodates it over time. He suspected this might have been the case for me, since I'd presented with limited symptoms, and because of the way the tumor pressed up against my liver, it appeared it might have been there for quite some time.

My mind flashed back through the past several years, imagining how things might have been different if we had caught it sooner and wondering how long it might have been growing inside me. As much as I hated my body right now, it was fascinating how much it could handle and conceal.

Over the next twenty minutes, I volleyed question after question from my list to Dr. Swami, asking about everything from whether surgery would be an option and what treatments he would recommend to what had caused the cancer. They were nearly impossible to answer without a biopsy and more information, but he was a good sport and very patiently took time to answer each.

He was unable to know with any degree of certainty whether surgery could be an option, but his gut feeling was that the spots in my liver could be adenomas, and if they were, that would mean the kidney cancer was still localized and we'd be able to operate—an opinion he shared while also trying to ensure I didn't get too far ahead of myself. I could tell he didn't want me to get attached to the idea of surgery, since we wouldn't know if it'd be possible until the biopsy came back and we had to make sure we ruled out any metastatic disease first. But surrounded by bad news everywhere I looked, I clung tight to this tiny sliver of hope.

The idea of moving forward with systemic treatment instead of surgery was a thought that tortured me. Everyone who knew about my diagnosis kept asking when I was going to have surgery, and when I searched through support groups, I noticed the majority of the other patients had all had their tumors removed. The team at Huntsman wanted to be careful, since in some cases it could be important to start treatment as soon as possible instead of heading to surgery if the cancer had spread. At the time, the thought of not removing it felt like far more than leaving the cancer behind; it felt like they were leaving *me* behind. I must have replayed that section of the audio from the appointment a hundred times in the days leading up to my MRI, looking for the light at the end of the tunnel, hoping he'd be right and they could operate.

As we made our way through all the questions on my list, we came across one of my most pressing, which I had been actively avoiding in an attempt to hold my composure. My voice began to crack and the emotion took over as I hesitantly asked, "What happens if it has spread? What's my prognosis?" This question was a double-edged sword. I wanted to know what I was dealing with, but I also didn't know if I had the strength to stomach the answer.

I was again asking questions that he didn't have the answers for. There were so many variables at play, but he tried to provide me with any answers he could to help ease my worry and distress. We wouldn't know until we had more information, but in general, the new treatments for kidney cancer were much better than they'd been in the past, and some of the immunotherapies being tested were showing as many as 50 percent of patients still alive and on treatment a few years out from diagnosis, and the end points had not yet been reached. There was still hope.

I stared back down at my notebook. I had asked what felt like a million questions at this point, all of which seemed to share a common answer: "We don't know." I'd have to get used to those three words, as they'd soon follow me everywhere I went. Over the months and years to follow, the response to nearly every question in my case would be followed by "we don't know." The uncertainty often left me feeling both scared and desperate. I'd spent my whole life planning five steps ahead, so this sudden adjustment to taking things day by day wasn't easy. I wouldn't be leaving the room with many answers that day, but at least for now we finally had a plan forward.

As the appointment wrapped up, Brian and I walked back down the same hallway we'd come in, but before reaching the door, we were directed over to the scheduler to get us on the books for my MRI, biopsy, and follow-up appointment in the coming weeks. I took a seat on the other side of the plexiglass window, and Brian stood behind me. The woman at the window appeared distracted as she asked for my name and kept an ear to the conversation between her coworkers as she pulled up my record. "It looks like we have you down for two MRIs and a biopsy." I nodded to confirm. She clicked a few buttons and pivoted in her chair to catch more of the conversation behind her, then swiveled back to the window. "All right, I've got you down for the twenty-seventh," she stated matter-of-factly.

Wait, what? That was three weeks away. If I couldn't get in for an MRI for three weeks, it'd be over a month from now before I could start treatment. That couldn't be right. The scheduler seemed a bit distracted; maybe she'd missed a note on my account. "That's three weeks away. You don't have anything sooner?" I asked.

"Nope, that's it," she responded back without a single further click. I wasn't sure how their systems worked, but it felt like she hadn't even checked. As I looked around, it wasn't just her; everyone seemed distracted, and my eyes started to fill with tears. I felt like I was falling through the cracks all over again. I needed to schedule these scans, and the results might quite literally spell out life or death for me. I didn't know how fast the cancer had been growing, but I'd heard of people who'd been taken by their cancer within a month, and with my limited understanding of cancer and my disease, I didn't know if I had a month to spare.

I asked one more time, "Are you sure? It sounded like the doctor wanted me to get in for the scans as soon as possible. Do you have anything sooner?" She looked slightly annoyed as she checked again. I felt like a burden. "If we separate them, we can get you in on the twenty-second and the twenty-seventh, but that's the earliest I can do."

I felt a tear silently slip from the corner of my eye. This wasn't how I'd expected today to go. Just a week ago when I left the ER, I'd found a small sense of comfort in feeling like we finally had answers and I'd have a team ready to help us figure this thing out. My new oncologist might not have answers yet, but I'd felt his empathy, compassion, and urgency. However, the moment I stepped out of the room, it felt like I was back at square one. Just another patient with a sad story, pushing for an appointment on an already full calendar. Back to being lost in a system that at the moment didn't really seem to care.

Feeling dejected, I took the appointment that at least got the abdominal MRI bumped up to two weeks instead of three and told myself I'd figure the rest out later. It was at that moment that I realized that as much as I hated making waves, learning to advocate for myself would have to become an active part of my care.

As we got up from the window and made our way back to the car, I tried to reconcile the emotions that had come over me. This had moved beyond sadness; these emotions were laced with bitterness, frustration, and fear. I feared what the delays might mean in terms of my care and the cancer that would be left unchecked inside me, but I also found myself bitter that I felt like I had to fight to be heard. Everyone had their own lives they could escape to, but I couldn't escape from mine. The emotions stewed as we began our drive home. I pulled out my phone as a distraction and was met with a wall of notifications. I scanned quickly through them and turned to Brian.

"Did you see there were protesters inside the Capitol?"

"There are protesters at the Capitol?" he replied, confused at why this would be news.

"No, protesters inside the Capitol. People are actually inside," I said as I began scanning through articles with pictures of people scaling the walls of the building. Had this been happening while we were at Huntsman? Suddenly, the distracted staff started to make a whole lot more sense, and I was hit with a wave of guilt. Here I was, worried about the cancer and feeling bad for myself, thinking that everyone seemed too distracted to care, but there were clearly much bigger things happening. It was the reality check I needed. Yes, the cancer might be destroying my life, but for everyone else, life went on, and people were just doing their best to make it through their own day. It was a pivotal moment for me that built a new perspective I'd learn to lean on in the months ahead. Life was bigger than any one moment or situation.

From that day forward, I acknowledged what little control I had on this journey. My life was dependent on and tightly coupled with the lives of hundreds of others, everyone from the phlebotomists and lab techs to the medical billers, doctors, nurses, and schedulers. Each one of them had their own life, problems, and priorities that existed outside the four walls that had brought us all together. The next time things went wrong, I'd challenge myself to put myself in their shoes first. To imagine their life and anything they might be dealing with themselves that could be influencing the situation and try to find little ways to make their lives easier if I could. If their day went better, likely so would mine, and we'd both be better off for it. I might be the one battling cancer, but I couldn't do it without their help. This was no longer just about me; this was we.

— 8 —

Sometimes I think I'm doing okay, then the next moment
I'm crying in the kitchen over chicken.
—Instagram post, January 9, 2021

T HE DAYS THAT followed my first appointment were just as trying as the ones that had preceded it. Everyone talks about the physical battle with cancer and the toll the treatments take on your body, but we don't often talk about the mental endurance it takes. The constant worry that occupies your mind, the emotions that sneak up on you at the most inopportune moments, learning to juggle these new obstacles while you schedule appointments, coordinate follow-ups, fight with insurance, and still try to hold down a full-time job so you don't lose said insurance. I still had all the same unanswered questions and unknowns from before but now had so much more work to do; over the next few weeks, I'd need to go for two MRIs, a biopsy, genetic screening, a surgery consult, and a colonoscopy. I'd also be researching cancer centers, locating institutions for second opinions, working full-time, and deciding if Brian and I would be keeping and following through with the house we were building. It all felt so overwhelming; each one of the tasks in isolation was stressful enough, but combined, they felt nearly impossible.

This window between when you find out that you might have cancer and the day you begin treatment is a special kind of hell I wouldn't wish on my worst enemy, and quite honestly, for me, it's one of the most difficult parts of having cancer. It's also why I advocate so strongly for supporting patients emotionally during this phase of their diagnosis. It doesn't matter the stage or type of cancer you're diagnosed with or where your treatment might ultimately lead you— the window between "you have cancer" and "we're actually doing something about it" is a time that can send anyone into a spiral.

I'd love to tell you I masterfully navigated through this phase of my diagnosis with ease, keeping all the balls in the air by tapping into the reservoir of "strength" everyone else seemed to find from within. With all of it behind me, I could sure paint a rosy picture and act as if it were my strength that powered me through these weeks, but that would just be a bold-faced lie. Nothing about this phase of my life was easy or natural, and I certainly never felt strong. I was in pure sur-vival mode, and folks, I limped through it. I wasn't a beacon of strength or inspiration but instead the poster child for "If you can't beat fear, just do it scared."

For most of my life, I had been the cautious one. My close, lifelong friend, Tanya, was always the risk taker between the two of us. As a kid, I envied her sense of adventure and carefree nature while I usually nervously stood on the side-lines, too overwhelmed by the risks and consequences to venture out of my comfort zone. And after a rough relation-ship and a severely traumatizing event in my teens left me with a healthy dose of PTSD, I became a true recluse who feared everything in the world around me. You name it, I was scared of it. The last thing anyone would have labeled me was strong.

Which is why I found it a bit ironic when people made comments and began associating my journey with strength. Nothing about me had changed except I'd acquired a diagnosis that confirmed one of my greatest fears, and I'd spent the entire week after my diagnosis a swollen-eyed puddle of tears. This didn't feel like strength. Surely, if they saw the sheer amount of tissues I'd gone through in the last week, they'd retract their statements and think I was a fraud. However, over time, I came to define strength as not the absence of fear but instead a product of persevering through it.

My first chance to persevere through the fear would be a colonoscopy the day after my first oncology appointment. I was beyond nervous beforehand.

You might be thinking a colonoscopy is an odd thing to order for a workup on kidney cancer, and you'd be right; this definitely wasn't standard protocol. It was part of a workup I'd been going through a few weeks before I was diagnosed to track down the cause of the lower abdominal cramps I'd been dealing with. The new ob-gyn I'd been seeing suspected they might be endometriosis, but since the workup for that typically required an exploratory surgery, she'd put me in touch with a gastroenterologist, who'd ordered a colonoscopy to rule out a couple of other things first. Since that appointment was already on the books and we still weren't sure what the lesions in my liver were, they wanted me to keep the appointment to rule anything like colon cancer out.

So here I was with my two bottles of blue Gatorade, some Miralax powder, and a tether to the bathroom for the next twenty-four hours, preparing for my first sedated procedure. I wasn't quite sure what to expect. I'd heard horror stories about the prep. Even though I'd already checked with my doctor, I'd seen a warning for people with kidney disease on the Miralax powder and grew worried. Highlighting my lack of knowledge about nearly anything medically related at the time and being completely unaware of the difference between kidney disease and kidney cancer, I was worried about how my kidneys might handle it. I might have had a bone to pick with one of them; I really wanted to keep them both functioning.

I imagine the prep could be pretty miserable if you're out gallivanting around town, but working from home with quick access to a bathroom, it really wasn't that bad. The worst part was the anticipation for the next day that kept me up that night as my mind raced through the worst possible scenarios.

Although we were fairly confident we were dealing with kidney, not colon, cancer, I was still nervous about what they might find. I mean, we hadn't thought an ultrasound would find a gigantic tumor on my kidney either, and yet here we were.

The next morning, Brian dropped me at the front entrance of the same hospital where we'd found the cancer. As I glanced over toward the ER, my stomach sank as I remembered all that'd transpired there just a week prior. The heightened emotion, mixed in with nerves and an empty stomach, made me feel nauseous as I navigated the halls of the hospital to the clinic in the basement of the building.

By the time they wheeled me back to the procedure room, I was a nervous wreck. It all felt so surreal as I looked up at the room around me. At twenty-nine, I'd thought I'd be preparing for pregnancy, not a colonoscopy; I didn't belong here. I felt a tear slip from the corner of my eye as the doctor, Dr. Sossenheimer, entered the room. He introduced himself as he washed his hands in the sink behind me and talked me through the procedure. He must have sensed the nerves in my voice, and as he finished, he came around to the side of the bed to check on me. "You seem a little nervous. How are you doing?" he asked in a concerned and gentle tone. My appointment started about an hour late, so I knew he'd already been running behind schedule, but he made an intentional pause to focus on me in that moment, as if neither time nor anything else mattered. I didn't know what it was about it, but it struck me to my core; it felt like he genuinely cared.

That's all it took, and the floodgates opened. I felt the tears stream down my face as I began to share with him my nerves not only about the procedure itself but also my fears of what they might find. His eyes softened as he crouched down next to the bed to be at eye level. "I can understand why you're scared. You've been through a lot the last few days, but I don't want you to worry. You're in good hands, and we're not going to let anything happen to you."

The tears began to let up as my trust in him grew and I felt the compassion in his voice. I nodded as he continued. "I saw your scans, and I know you're worried about what's in your liver. We don't know what this is yet, but we're going to figure it out together. It may not seem like it now, but regardless of what lies ahead, you've been given a gift to see the world through a new perspective. One that not many have the chance to experience."

He wiped a tear from my cheek before giving a few final words of encouragement. "Remember, we're going to be right here the whole time. You're in good hands, and we're not going to let anything happen to you," he reiterated as he stood up. Both the anesthesiologist and medical assistant provided words of encouragement as the medication to put me under entered my line. The last thing I remembered was the medical tech, who squeezed my hand and told me he'd be praying for me as my eyes grew heavy and I drifted off.

Over the next few days, I reflected on the words shared with me before the procedure. That moment was truly one of the most genuine and real interactions I'd ever had with a doctor. But I couldn't help but sit and ponder what exactly he'd meant when he said I'd been given a gift to see the world through a new perspective. I didn't feel like cancer was a gift. So far, it kind of sucked, and I'd never asked for a new perspective. I kind of liked the one I already had. At the time, this gift felt like one I desperately wished I could return. However, the words he used in that moment meant far less to me than the sincerity he shared them with, which is what I chose to focus on instead. But over time, I'd truly come to appreciate that advice and realize just how right he'd been about the perspective my diagnosis would one day bring me.

Just as Dr. Sossenheimer's words would grow with me over time, so would my gratitude and appreciation for these moments and even for the fear I carried with me through them. In the weeks that followed, I'd have many more interactions just like this, where I'd be doing well, feeling proud of myself for holding it together, before I'd suddenly crumble and fall apart again. I felt like a burden every time, but when I look back with hindsight, I can see true beauty in these interactions. And I'm left with a plethora of memories of normal, everyday people taking a second out of their busy lives to pause and spend a moment with a perfect stranger—offering comfort and sharing vulnerable stories of their own. If you'd given me a chance at the time, I would have done anything to suppress those fears, but looking back now, I wouldn't trade those interactions for the world, and I cherish them deeply. They're my reminder of the good in people, and they laid the foundation for how I'd eventually build my own definition of strength. I'll always remember and cherish the memories with all of these wonderful strangers who helped build that strength with me.

— 9 —

These results will likely tell us if I'm stage 4 or if we've caught it before it's spread. So join me today and tomorrow putting all the positive energy and prayers we can in for good news! Benign growths and no spread is what we want!!
—Instagram post, January 11, 2021

"YOU NEVER TRULY appreciate what you have until it's gone." We've all likely come across some variation of this phrase before, usually found in bold lettering plastered on top of a mountainesque backdrop meant to invoke inspiration and meaning. Before my diagnosis, these quotes and phrases would often inspire reflections on missed opportunities, but post-diagnosis, they evolved into much more. Through the events that would transpire after my diagnosis and through treatment, this phrase would leave me reflecting on the strength of our bodies, the privilege of good health, and the very essence of life itself. Which sounds like its own dose of inspirational mumbo jumbo, but after a few scares, close calls, and a bumpy ride on the cancer coaster, quite honestly, nothing else rings truer.

My first bump on that coaster and the first reminder of just how fragile life is came for me on biopsy day, when a quick routine procedure cascaded into a series of events that led to my first hospital admission and brought me a new appreciation of the resilience of the human body.

I'd originally only been scheduled for a kidney biopsy, but when the MRI was unable to rule out the spots in my liver as benign lesions, they decided to do a biopsy of the liver at the same time. When the day finally arrived, I was a bundle of nerves. In the days leading up to the procedure, I'd gone for both my MRIs and a surgery consult. The surgeon I'd met with was confident he could remove the kidney tumor but advised it'd only be worth it if those spots in my liver didn't end up being metastatic disease. A recent study published suggested that removing the primary tumor (the one on my kidney) once a patient was already stage four didn't improve their overall survival. Even though there have continued to be studies investigating this since and it's not a closed case, the study was practice changing at the time, as up until that point, it was common for patients to have a nephrectomy—their kidney removed—prior to starting treatment. This explained why I saw so many other patients in the support groups who'd had theirs removed. The study argued that due to the lack of improvement in outcomes for many patients, it was better not to operate so you didn't have to put patients through surgery and could begin treatment sooner.

As the surgeon described the study, I understood the logic behind it but I was sorely disappointed. Now that I knew the tumor was there, it was constantly on my mind. I couldn't stop torturing myself by touching it, tracing its outline with my hand, surveying for growth, and trying to figure out how long it might have been there. It was a constant reminder of the uncertainty we faced and the storm brewing overhead. I wanted this thing out, and the one thing standing between me and that surgery was this biopsy.

The appointment for my procedure was scheduled for ten AM, and I arrived at nine thirty to complete the paperwork in hopes it might lead to them calling me back sooner. I'd learn that arriving early is a rather futile effort in health care. Instead, it only led to me waiting in the lobby for over an hour, killing time alone. I'd brought one of my favorite books to keep me distracted during the wait but found myself rereading the same paragraph over and over while my mind wandered. So instead I took to texting Brian, who was in the parking lot, and he kept me loaded up with a steady stream of cute dog videos and funny TikToks to keep me busy.

As I watched other patients slowly clear out of the room, called back one by one, I wondered if they were missing something from me or if there was a step I hadn't completed. I was getting ready to stand up to check in with the front desk when a text from my dad flashed across my screen. Heard this song this morning and thought of you, he said, offering a link to a video of Bob Marley's "Three Little Birds." I opened the link, and my headphones filled with a familiar tune. *Don't you worry about a thing . . .* I let the song play out as my eyes filled with tears. My dad wanted to tell me that everything was going to be all right.

I've always looked up to my dad, and he's one of the few people on this planet who I feel understands me in a way no one else does, without a single word spoken. I knew exactly what the video meant and felt as if he were waiting there with me. I closed my eyes and let the song loop until my name was called.

Once I was finally called back, the nurse handed me a gown that I swear to this day is still the only gown I've ever seen fully intact. I changed into the limited-edition gem and zoned in on the snowflake-like pattern printed across the fabric as the nurse started my IV. "You nervous?" she asked, placing the pulse ox on my finger and watching my heart rate go for a sprint.

"Very," I replied.

She smirked and told me not to worry as she queued up the medications, which she assured me would take care of the nerves soon enough. Unlike my colonoscopy, they'd need me alert for the biopsy so I could follow breathing instructions.

Which meant I'd be awake through the entire procedure. This sounded like literal torture, and I contemplated if it was too late to back out just as a young doctor entered the room.

He introduced himself as Dr. Hartness, the "fellow" who would be completing the biopsies, and began walking me through what to expect.

I had no idea what a fellow was. *What an odd way to refer to himself,* I thought as I tried to gauge his age while my nerves mounted and I admittedly began questioning his experience. I knew liver biopsies were more complicated, and he couldn't have been much older than I was, which made me wonder just how many of these he could possibly have done. Looking back now at these interactions sure makes me wish I'd caught a few episodes of a medical drama or two before I was diagnosed. Even the slightest knowledge of the structure of the medical system sure would have been nice context to have in these situations.

For anyone else who may be missing the same context, here's a quick rundown. The hierarchy in care starts with medical students who aren't doctors yet and who spend four years in medical school. Upon graduation, they become interns, which is their title during their first year in practical training, where they work under the supervision of more senior medical personnel. Next is residency, which lasts two to seven years, depending on the resident's specialty. Residents are doctors who have completed their internship and are gaining specialized experience in a particular field of medicine under the supervision of attending physicians. Once they are finished with residency, some doctors will go directly into practice; others will continue on with a fellowship, which can last one to three years, depending on the subspecialty, to acquire more advanced skills and knowledge. Then finally, you have attending physicians, who are fully qualified and independent doctors who have completed all training stages. They are capable of supervising medical students, interns, residents, and fellows.

Dr. Hartness began walking me through the procedure, which would be completed in a two-part process. We'd start with the biopsy of my kidney, where I'd lie flat on my stomach, and they'd access the tumor through my back. After that was complete, they'd have me roll over, and we'd do the same thing for the largest lesion in my liver. Then, once they had all the samples they needed, I'd be sent to a recovery area, where they'd have me lie flat for a few hours to prevent a bleed, and I'd be discharged shortly thereafter.

After consenting to the procedure, I got positioned on the bed, and the nurse called the attending into the room. Still oblivious as to who an attending was, I barely acknowledged him as he walked in. I'd already begun my ritual of zoning out, with my head down and eyes closed, silently trying to get a handle on the nerves. He lighthearted and endearingly chuckled at the lack of acknowledgment. Attending physicians are often used to answering and handling the big questions before any procedure. Had I known that's who he was, my inquisitive nature would have thrown several at him. So my lack of acknowledgement, I'm sure, was out of the norm, like standing next to the league all-star while asking the newly drafted recruit for training tips. He gave the go-ahead to the nurse to begin, who flushed my IV and pushed in the medication. I felt the effects almost instantly as my anxiety dropped from a ten to a three.

I didn't know what to expect. Honestly, I thought I'd feel a bit high, maybe a little drowsy, but I was surprised that cognitively I didn't really feel a whole lot different. I was still aware of everything around me, and my train of thought was uninterrupted. All the anxious thoughts were still there, but it was like someone had shut off the valve to caring. When I felt a quick prick of the needle to deliver the local anesthetic, my panic was replaced by apathy—a shift from "Oh my god, this is happening" to a casual acknowledgment of the circumstances.

I had to hold as still as physically possible and follow the breathing instructions as they came to ensure my liver didn't move while they took the sample. I'd settled into an odd position for my head, which I regretted, as my neck was feeling pinched, but I was locked in. Using an ultrasound as his guide, the doctor located the target, and it was time to begin. He instructed me to take a deep breath and hold as he inserted the needle. I wondered when I'd feel the pressure they'd informed me was coming, but before I knew it, it was already over. I didn't feel a thing.

That was anticlimactic, I thought as I heard them transfer the sample over to the pathologists in the room to confirm they had snagged enough tissue. They confirmed they had a positive sample, and the doctor wrapped things up from there. They cleaned and bandaged the area before instructing me to carefully roll over onto my back so they could begin the liver biopsy. I rolled to my side, then cautiously onto my back, as if it were made of glass, and got resettled. I opened my eyes and watched as they cleaned and prepped an area at the bottom of my sternum, the bone that connects your rib cage in the center of your chest.

I was curious to watch the procedure, something I knew my nerves would never allow me to stomach on my own. But I wondered if the IV liquid courage coursing through my veins just might do the trick. I tucked my chin in, cranked my head down, and began watching as they injected the local anesthetic before suddenly, the anxiety rushed back in and hit me like a tidal wave. Hard pass. I stared back up at the ceiling tiles as they marked their entry point.

I was hoping the liver biopsy would be just as painless as the kidney, but unfortunately, I wasn't quite as lucky. I felt the pressure as he pressed down on the needle, piercing my skin as I let out an involuntary "Ope!" as if I were a midwesterner trying to squeeze past someone in the market. I tried to convince myself the pain was just "a little pressure" as I looped more calming affirmations in my head. I felt him push down farther, grabbing the biopsy before coming back out. I thought we might be done, but then he went back in one more time. This time, that little pressure turned into a sharp pain and the midwesterner came out again, this time slightly more agitated.

"Ope, ouch, oh okay, yep, I felt that one," I said, grimacing through the pain as the needle plunged down and quickly back out again. The sharp pain quickly dissipated, and I heard the chatter as they sent the sample back across the room to our pathologist friends for confirmation.

"Looks good," they confirmed. The doctor cleaned and covered the area, then gave the all clear for them to head back to the lab. He did a final check with the ultrasound to ensure there wasn't a bleed, then that was it; just like that, we were done. I couldn't believe I'd actually made it through it. Maybe it wasn't all that bad after all. I let out a big sigh of relief.

"You did great," the doctor confirmed as he walked me through the next steps. Someone would come by shortly to take me up to the recovery area. He pointed to the biopsy location for my liver and told me I'd have two small bandages covering the very small incisions at each of the biopsy sites that should heal up quickly, but I'd need to keep them dry and avoid baths for two weeks. Which, since I was a "bath person," sounded like it would be the worst part of this thing. I thanked both Dr. Hartness and the attending, Dr. Shaaban, as they gave me well wishes and headed out the door.

As I waited for a transporter to take me back to the recovery area, I started to feel an ache in my right shoulder. "I don't feel very well," I notified the nurse as she began putting away the blood pressure cuff and tools they'd used for the procedure.

"You don't feel well?" she repeated, undeterred from her task as she continued to pull drawers and pack away the room.

"No, I have a bit of pain, and I don't know . . . I don't feel very well," I replied timidly, trying to sort out a better description as the nausea set in and a bead of sweat slipped from my forehead.

"Yeah, you just had a couple biopsies. You'll probably be a little sore for a few days," she reassured me.

She wasn't taking me seriously. This didn't feel normal. "No, I really don't feel well," I reiterated in a more escalated tone, the panic slipping through my voice as I began to feel lightheaded. I begged her to help me take off my socks as I began overheating and the lightheadedness sank in. "Can you please get the doctor?" I pleaded.

The panic in my voice had finally caught her attention, and she called for the doctor to come back in as I frantically tossed blankets off me to cool down. My palms began to sweat and my vision narrowed as the doctor entered the room. He asked what I was feeling, and I mentioned the pain I was having in my right shoulder.

"Your right shoulder?" he asked, sounding a little concerned.

"Yes, it's not a sharp pain, it's radiating," I confirmed. The pain felt familiar. It was reminiscent of the pain I'd had after a laparoscopy surgery to remove my gallbladder in my teens. The pain is usually caused by the gas from the procedure. I didn't think they'd used any gas—these weren't laparoscopy incisions—but I wondered if it could still be related and normal.

"Get an ultrasound back on her," Dr. Shaaban instructed with urgency as Dr. Hartness and a few nurses shuffled back into the room. "I think I'm going to pass out," I muttered softly as my head fell back and my vision faded.

I felt a blood pressure cuff wrap tightly around my left arm. "Her blood pressure is crashing," the nurse called out with urgency in her voice. "Fifty-nine over thirty-six."

"There's a bleed," I heard from one of the doctors in quick succession as the organized chaos kicked off around me. I was slipping in and out of consciousness as I struggled to keep my eyes open. This was my biggest fear, and here we were. It was actually happening. It didn't feel like real life; this was the kind of thing that happened in medical dramas and TV shows, the ones I avoided, not to me. My eyes grew heavy.

"I don't feel well . . . ," I whispered softly, trailing off as I struggled to verbalize the words.

"Elevate her legs," someone called out as Dr. Hartness swooped and lifted them into what felt like an angled fetal position. My head now pointed down, the blood rushing to my brain.

"Stay with me," he said as I fought off the ever-growing urge to close my eyes. "Don't close your eyes, stay with me, we're right here," he kept reminding and reassuring me as he continued to hold my legs as everyone worked around him.

I could collectively feel their adrenaline as their training kicked in, and I heard the uneasiness in their voices. I felt utterly helpless as I used every ounce of energy I had to hold my eyes open. There was nothing I could do.

A nurse moved to the phone on the wall behind me. "Should I call her husband?" she asked.

I watched as she nervously dialed his number, and I tried to decode the worry etched on her face. A wave of fear and uncertainty washed over me as I began to wonder if this was what it was like to die. Surely, these kinds of things happened all the time. It was just a complication. I was going to be fine . . . right?

I could hear the sounds of the medical team working on me and the urgent voices of the doctor's request to move me to CT.

After a couple rings, I listened as the nurse connected with Brian on the other line. "Your wife had a small complication during the procedure, and we think you should come in," she explained, giving him brief instructions to head to the recovery area where I'd meet him after a scan to check the status of the bleed. Which is where my memory briefly fades out.

The next thing I remember, doctors were rushing me through the halls of the hospital to CT for an emergency scan. As we waited in the hallway, I could feel the tension in the air.

I could sense the doctors' concern as the rush and adrenaline slowed and the silence became palpable.

At this point, I was in a decent amount of pain. The radiating pain in my right shoulder had turned into a sharp, stabbing pain in my upper abdomen that'd course through my body with the slightest movement but could still be avoided if I managed to hold perfectly still. Which worked well until it came time to be loaded onto the scanner.

When it became available, they wheeled me into the room, the doctor graciously thanking his colleague for squeezing us in, and they helped me onto the machine—a tricky maneuver while attempting to stay horizontal. I felt a sharp pain as we made the transfer, then I began to feel a cramping in my lower abdomen. It too felt familiar, and I tried to place the sensation. It was reminiscent of the painful cramps I'd been getting for the last year and a half before my period each month. This feeling was identical to that pain but at a lower intensity, sitting at a four instead of a ten, uncomfortable but not unbearable. I would find out later that this pain was caused by the blood draining into my pelvis.

After completing the scan, I was loaded back onto the hospital bed and moved into a recovery room, where Brian waited for me. He was sitting on a chair next to the bed, bouncing his leg and nervously awaiting my arrival. I couldn't have been more relieved to see him. I wanted to tell him everything that'd just transpired or even just how grateful I was to have him there, but I knew I wouldn't be able to get through the tears. The bleed in my liver had agitated my diaphragm and made it painful to breathe. I knew crying would only make it worse. I let him know I wasn't ready to talk quite yet as they began transferring me onto the bed.

I tried to place my arms behind me and lift with my legs to crab-walk my way off one bed and onto the other to make the transfer on my own, but the pain was excruciating, and my arms buckled beneath me. It felt as if there were a hundred knives in my upper abdomen trying to twist and stab their way out with the slightest movement. The pain was so sudden and sharp that it'd ripple through the rest of my body before slowly disappearing, almost convincing me it was gone until the next time I moved. I was unable to make the transfer on my own, so a few nurses used a sheet to drag first the top of my body onto the bed, then my lower half until I was fully situated. Which ultimately might have been more painful than moving myself as they tugged, pulled, and scooched me over.

Once I was positioned in the new bed, a nurse grabbed my vitals, drew a vial of blood, and hung a bag of fluids before leaving the room, letting me know she'd be back to check on me shortly. As she left, I looked back down at Brian, my eyes once again filling with tears.

"It's okay, I'm right here. We can talk whenever you're ready, or we can just sit here. I'm not going anywhere."

I couldn't have imagined a better way for him to support me in that moment. It was exactly what I needed. I needed the silence to talk myself through the pain and to process everything that had just happened, but I needed and craved the comfort of having him there as well. His reassurance and presence meant more than words ever could.

Trying to provide a distraction and a change of subject before the emotions resurfaced, he grabbed the remote from the bed. "Anything I can put on for you?" he asked as he began flipping through the channels until landing on *The Office*, one of our favorite shows.

"That's good," I told him.

"*The Office* it is." He turned up the volume a few notches to drown out the noise of the busy hospital but ensured that it was still quiet enough so I could think. Our marriage was so new and hadn't been tested in this way before. I didn't know how he so naturally knew all the right things to do and say. I could see the worry in his eyes, but his actions never let it show.

Brian and I sat comfortably in silence until we heard a knock at the door. I looked over my shoulder to find Dr. Hartness walking into the room. He introduced himself to Brian, then stood at the end of the bed to check in and chat with us both. He appeared calm and relaxed, which was a drastic shift from all the commotion we'd experienced together just a few hours earlier. I figured at least this must be a good sign.

He let us know that the scans showed a small bleed that had come from the biopsy site in the liver but that it appeared to be slowing or have stopped on its own, since my blood pressure had stabilized and the most recent labs they'd drawn showed a slowing in the blood loss. Which was good news. It meant that I shouldn't need surgery or anything to stop the bleeding. Instead, they'd just monitor and keep an eye on me for another hour or two to ensure the trend held before sending me home.

He stayed and chatted with Brian and me for a while before heading out and letting us know he'd be back to check in one more time before they discharged me. Since it didn't look like I'd need surgery, I asked if I could graduate from the sponge on a stick I'd been provided to keep my mouth wet to a glass of water, since we didn't need to worry about the food or drink restriction for anesthesia. I hadn't been allowed to eat or drink anything up to this point, and the edges of my mouth had become sticky and dry. He laughed, said he'd put the orders in, and let the nurse know on his way out.

The next time the nurse came back around, I got not only a glass of water but even juice with a cup full of ice. I was really living the high life. Brian poured the juice into the cup and handed it to me before we both realized I was supposed to stay lying flat. I tried to lift my head up and crunch up toward the cup but felt a sharp pain as I engaged the muscles in my stomach. Hmm . . . this was going to be a bit tricky. Brian grabbed a straw, and we tried again. This time I moved the cup up near my shoulder and moved my head to the straw instead, keeping the rest of my body perfectly still. Success! I felt the cold juice hit my tongue as I savored its sweetness. I didn't drink sugary drinks or juices very often, so the sweetness was both overwhelming and wonderfully addicting. Before I knew it, I'd downed the entire glass. Which soon would become a problem.

About twenty minutes after downing that prized apple juice, I realized I needed to use the bathroom—a mild sensation at first that I tried to ignore. I'd be out of here soon enough. I could make it, I told myself. However, the bag of fluid and two beverages I'd downed had other plans. The urgency grew until I knew if I held it any longer, we were going to have a problem on our hands. The nurse informed me the bathroom was down the hall, so I'd need to get up so we could walk down there together. "Get up? I thought I had to lay flat for a few hours?" I asked, confused.

"No, you should be fine. I can help you get up, and we can walk down there if you really need to go," she insisted.

That didn't seem right. Everything I'd read leading up to the biopsy to prepare myself and the few other patients I'd chatted with beforehand had all emphasized the need to lie flat after the procedure for several hours to prevent a bleed. I'd already had a bleed, so this seemed like a bad idea.

I asked again, "Are you sure?"

Sounding slightly more annoyed this time, she said she'd check my chart to see if there were any instructions that said I couldn't stand, but if I needed to use the restroom, it was down the hall. I'd need to either get up or I'd have to use a bedpan. She walked over to the computer, and I heard a few clicks from the mouse as I sensed her irritation. "Nope, no notes. You should be fine to stand," she confirmed.

This didn't feel right, and I could hardly move, but I didn't exactly want to use a bedpan in front of my husband either. "Okay, I'll try to stand up," I decided.

She pulled down the guardrail on the side of the bed so I could roll my legs over. I couldn't even adjust myself in the bed without intense pain. I knew this was not going to be fun. I took a deep breath to prepare myself, only to remember the pain breathing deeply brought in itself. I took a few small shallow breaths instead to build my courage as I positioned my right arm behind me and began to push myself up.

"No, no, no! Ooooo, no, that HURTS!" I involuntarily cried out in pain, quickly lowering myself back down to the bed. The excruciating, stabbing pain that radiated from my abdomen was by far the worst the pain had been. "I can't do it, I can't get up," I said, defeated.

"Do you really want to use a bedpan?" the nurse asked, her tone filled with judgment. Of course I didn't *want* to use a bedpan. I didn't want everyone in the room to watch me use it, and I certainly didn't want her to have to deal with it either, so I decided to make one more attempt. If I moved more quickly this time, the pain might be more intense getting up, but once I got into a sitting position, maybe I could breathe through it. I just needed to make it all the way up. I counted down in my head as I prepared myself—three . . . two . . . one . . . I pushed as hard as I could off the bed, hoping one strong push would do the trick.

The pain on the way up had nearly taken my breath away, but it got the job done. I was now sitting on the edge of the bed, my legs dangling over the side as I tried to catch my breath and get control of the pain. After a minute or two at the side of the bed, I'd finally recouped enough to give standing a try next. I counted again, this time out loud. "One . . . two . . . three . . . ," I said as I bit down on my lip, held my breath (big mistake), and groaned through the pain. That was it, I was standing . . . I was in excruciating pain, but I was standing.

The nurse encouraged me to step forward and begin walking with her. I didn't feel ready but stepped forward anyway, grasping tightly, locked around her arms. I took one step and started to feel dizzy again; all the same sensations I had been feeling a few hours prior came rushing back. I stopped. "I can't do this; I don't feel well," I said as I tried to reclaim my balance and the room started to spin.

"You're okay, just breathe through it." I'd already seen how this one played out. I was not going to simply breathe my way through this one.

"I can't," I replied, the panic escalating in my voice as the lightheadedness returned.

"Yes you can, just take a deep breath." Her tone was reminiscent of the nurse I'd interacted with earlier who thought I was overreacting. She called another nurse into the room to help.

"No, I literally can't," I said as I grimaced and moaned through the pain. "I can't take a deep breath, like physically. I can't." Growing frustrated as I felt my palms beginning to sweat again, I stepped back and lowered myself onto the bed. "I'm going to pass out," I warned.

She looked slightly annoyed until I started to fall back, and she tried to catch me while simultaneously sweeping my legs back up. I heard the Velcro of the blood pressure cuff peel back; my vision narrowed, and my eyes became heavy again. "Her blood pressure's dropping," I heard the new nurse at my side report back as a new chaotic frenzy ensued. They began stuffing pillows under my legs to elevate them and get the blood rushing back to my head again.

I caught a glimpse of Brian out of the corner of my eye, whose strong, silent facade cracked. "She told you she didn't feel well. She told you she was going to pass out!" He raised his voice in frustration that they had not listened to me sooner. I watched him in the background as they worked, and he looked on helplessly.

The next few minutes were a blur as they worked to get me stabilized. Once my blood pressure began to rise and the commotion slowed, the nurse left the room to notify and update the doctors. And I was left with one burning question on my mind: How in the world had this happened again, and why couldn't I get anyone to take me seriously? This clearly was a theme, and the common denominator at this point seemed to be me.

— 10 —

*The last 48 hours were pretty terrifying to be honest.
I always want to be completely transparent about my
journey, so I'm choosing to share all the details. Even the
embarrassing, gross and scary bits.*
—Instagram post, January 16, 2021*

A FTER I'D NEARLY passed out again, the doctors decided
to send me back for another scan to check if there was
another bleed. When we got back to the room, I knew there
was no way around it; I was going to be forced to get friendly
with that bedpan. I was still unable to stand, and my bladder was about to explode. I must say, there are few things
more humbling than sitting on top of a hollow metal basin to
relieve your bladder while the entire room looks on. The cold
stainless steel casing reminded me of something you'd see in
a prison cell, which felt rather fitting, as I felt both tortured
and trapped as the two nurses and Brian looked on. There was
something truly dehumanizing about losing the ability to care
for my most basic needs that left me feeling like both a burden
and a failure.

As the nurse left the room, I lay in silence, staring at the
ceiling and ruminating on the embarrassment until I heard a
gentle knock at the door. I glanced over my shoulder to see Dr.
Shaaban and Dr. Hartness enter the room. This was the first
time I'd seen Dr. Shaaban, the attending, since he'd escorted
me through the halls of the hospital. I studied his face as I

tried to connect the calm man in front of me to the one calling the shots in the commotion a few hours prior. He was a middle-aged man with olive skin, a salt-and-pepper goatee, and kind eyes that made me feel safe in his presence.

He updated us on the results of the latest scan, letting us know the bleed was slowing and my labs were stable. Since I was still unable to stand on my own, they had decided to admit me for the night for monitoring, but it might be a little while before they could find me a room. I wasn't surprised; we were in the middle of a COVID surge, and beds were difficult to come by, but I wasn't worried about how long I had to wait. I was just grateful to have more time to recover, since heading home to our three-story townhome and attempting to make it up the stairs to our bedroom sounded impossible.

After sharing the update, Dr. Shaaban and Dr. Hartness lingered in the room making small talk. Their schedules had been cleared for the day, so they were unrushed as they chatted with Brian and me.

"Have you always lived in the area?" Dr. Shaaban asked, transitioning the conversation.

"I grew up here but spent most of my twenties in Texas. I've been back for a little over a year but still haven't gotten used to the snow again. I hate the cold," I shared.

Dr. Shaaban laughed. "I'm originally from Egypt. While I enjoy the four seasons here, I don't care for the snow much either."

The four of us laughed and chatted, continuing to converse leisurely about what Brian and I did for a living and places we'd lived, in a moment that felt like a portal to another world. One where we were getting to know new friends outside the walls of a hospital as we all completely ignored the bed I was lying in or the fact that I'd let these two strangers stab me with big fancy needles a few hours prior.

Other than the brief moment I'd had with the gastroenterologist before my colonoscopy, I'd never had an interaction like this with a doctor. There always seemed to be a giant wall between me and the physician on the other side of the room, someone I'd be forced to entrust my life to without knowing anything about them. Which feels unnatural in a world where we can learn almost anything about those we interact with through social media.

As they began to feel more approachable, my trust in them grew. It made me wonder how different interactions with physicians, in general, might be if we were granted more time with them.

As I'd started to feel more like I was conversing with peers than doctors, I decided to ask them a few burning questions I had on my mind but had been too intimidated to ask. I wanted to learn about the language listed in my radiology report from my CT scan in the ER. I'd read the report about a hundred times at this point, and I'd discussed it with other patients in support groups, but the reports in general felt like they were written in a different language.

Mine had suggested that my tumor was likely chromophobe kidney cancer or an oncocytoma. Both of these were more rare than other types of kidney tumors, each accounting for about five percent of renal tumors each year, and they both typically carried a better prognosis. Oncocytomas were known to be benign, and chromophobe kidney cancer (ChRCC) became metastatic in only about five to ten percent of cases. This initially had made me hopeful, until I learned that if ChRCC does spread, it can be less likely to respond to the current treatments, which can negate the survival benefit.

I wondered why the radiologist had suggested it could be either of these from a scan, since most of what I'd read online said it was impossible to distinguish between types of kidney cancer from imaging. I'd also talked to several patients diagnosed with ChRCC, none of whom ever had it described in their scan prior to removal, so I took this opportunity to ask. "I actually had a question about one of my reports. In the report from my CT scan, at the end it mentioned it was possible to be an oncocytoma or chromophobe RCC. Did either of you read that in the report or know why they would have written it? I haven't found it in other reports."

Dr. Shaaban nodded his head as he began to reply. "Yes. I was actually the one who reviewed your scans and who made the note."

"Oh, really?" I replied, surprised. I still didn't know much about medicine but was surprised the same doctor overseeing my biopsy would have also been reading my scans. "Can you tell the type from imaging?" I inquired further.

"Not conclusively," he replied. "Which is why after reviewing your MRI yesterday, I suggested both a liver and a kidney biopsy today." He paused briefly, glancing at me in the bed with an expression washing over his face that looked like he might be questioning if he had made the right call, given the predicament I now found myself in. He refocused and continued, "Oncocytomas can have unique features that make them stand out on imaging. Specifically, a large central scar in the middle, which is something yours has. Chromophobe can occasionally have them too. Chromophobe renal cell carcinoma also can present with larger tumors and in patients slightly younger than the typical demographic for the more common types of kidney cancer. Oncocytomas are benign and chromophobe RCC doesn't spread very often, which is why it was important to biopsy the liver lesions to see if they are related or not. Some young women, especially those who have been on birth control, can have benign spots in their liver that may look like tumors. So we needed to test them to be sure."

I remembered seeing the scar he was describing at my first appointment when my oncologist pulled up my scans. I had no idea what I was looking at; the images looked just like blobs in different shades of black and white. But I remembered seeing a large mass in the middle that looked like it had been hit by an asteroid, leaving behind markings like craters in the moon. I didn't know what organ that was at the time, but the pieces were slowly beginning to fit together.

I continued to ask a million follow-up questions as I hung on Dr. Shaaban's every word, absorbing as much as I could. I wondered how I could be so utterly fascinated by my case medically and completely devastated by it at the same time. I appreciated how well he explained everything in easy-to-understand terms and how willing he was to entertain my questions, including those about how often he'd seen this before and how many patients experienced complications like I just had. He was honest and transparent, admitting this was the first time in over a twenty-year career he'd ever had a patient have a reaction like mine. They'd seen bleeds, but he'd never actually admitted a patient before. Guess there is a first for everything, but I think we both could have done without that first being today.

"How long will it take to get the results back from the biopsies?" I asked as we neared the end of the conversation.

"It'll be about a week," Dr. Shaaban replied, "but I promise I'll follow up with my colleagues daily to get the results back as soon as possible so we can get this figured out for you."

I appreciated his reassurance. It felt personal and real. We wrapped up the conversation just as he was called out of the room. I thanked him for his time before he stepped away, and he promised to be back to check in before he left for the evening.

As he stepped out of the room, Dr. Hartness, who'd been standing just a few feet away against the wall, moved in closer and rested his hand on the railing of the bed. "Wow, that was incredible . . . I want you to know just how special that was," he said with a profound look in his eyes, clearly moved.

I looked back at him, a bit perplexed. "What was?" I asked as I tried to retrace the conversation in case I'd missed something.

"All of it," he said. "That was an incredibly special moment to witness. Dr. Shaaban is an expert in imaging; he has written textbooks describing the very characteristics he described to you. Hearing him explain it back to a patient and the dialogue you two had was truly amazing." He continued to explain with clear admiration in his voice. "This is why I came here to study under that man." We continued chatting as he waited with us to find out if they were able to find me a room, and after about twenty minutes, he too was pulled away but promised to be back with an update.

Later that night, a transporter arrived at the door, ready to take me over to Huntsman Cancer Institute. They'd finally found me a room. Both doctors walked with us to the elevator, and before parting ways, Dr. Shaaban told us he wouldn't be working the next day but that he wanted to stop by in the morning after he dropped his daughter off at school. I appreciated the concern he'd shown and how late he and Dr. Hartness had both stayed into the night, checking on me every few hours, as I was sure they both had families to return to. Despite having a complication from the procedure, I was grateful for their care as we parted ways and the elevator door closed behind us.

The journey from the main university hospital over to Huntsman was a rocky one as we went in and out of elevators and bumped into walls along the way. Every bump sent sharp pains. I winced around every corner, slightly irritated that we'd clipped so many walls. The bed drifted like an IKEA cart with a mind of its own. While I was sick of playing bumper cars, I was equally certain I wouldn't be able to do much better had I been the one driving.

I wasn't sure what to expect as we arrived at the room. I'd never been admitted to a hospital before, and my only point of reference at the time was TV and movies, which always showed patients sharing a room with a stranger and a curtain drawn as they both eavesdropped on each other's conversations. As an introvert who really values their own space, I thought that sounded like a nightmare, but I wasn't exactly in a position to be picky. However, as they wheeled me into the room, it was nothing like I'd imagined. Not only did I have my own room, but it looked more like a hotel than a hospital room. *Surely we can't be in the right place?* In the spacious room, there was an entertainment-center-like space in front of the bed, with canned lighting, a large TV, shelves, and nice wardrobe cabinetry. On the opposite wall, there was a whiteboard used to track important patient information and goals. Then at the far end of the room, there was a cushy hospital reclining chair positioned next to a large window with a sitting bench overlooking the *U*—for the university—lit up on the mountainside. If I was going to be stuck in this bed all night, there were certainly worse places to be.

Brian helped me get settled in but wasn't able to stay. Since it was past visiting hours when we arrived, he hung out until my nurse came around to introduce herself knowing he would have to leave shortly thereafter. He got me tucked in with a warm blanket and plugged my phone to place it on the bedside table before saying his goodbyes. While I still hadn't mustered up the courage to talk about what had happened, simply having him there with me meant everything. What if something happened while he was gone? He wouldn't be in the parking lot this time to come to my rescue. A tear slipped from the corner of my eye. This would be the first night of our marriage we'd spent apart, and it wasn't going to be an easy one. He placed my phone beside me. "I'm just a call or text away, the whole night. It's going to be okay," he assured me as he kissed my forehead, squeezed my hand, and told me he loved me before reluctantly making his way to the door.

A few hours after he left, since I was unable to sleep, I grabbed my phone and began flipping through the pictures of smiling faces that filled my feed. The window into their lives was like a nice distraction from mine, but I found myself looking on with envy. Here I was, sipping on chicken broth and swapping out bedpans, while they were skiing down mountainsides. Why did my body have to fail me, and why hadn't I appreciated it while I could? I promised myself I'd never take my health for granted again if only I could get back to that state. It still hurt to breathe or even to move, something they told me might last a week or two as my body reabsorbed the blood but should get a little better each day. *I just need to get to tomorrow*, I reminded myself. *Tomorrow will be better than today*—a theme I'd lean on many times through the times ahead.

I didn't like the feelings that were surfacing as I watched the world continue on without me. The jealousy kept creeping in, no matter how much I tried to force it down. So I decided to put the phone away and write down my "one thing I'm grateful for" and "one thing I struggled with," then turned on the TV to wind down for the night. I flipped back and forth through the channels before eventually landing back on *The Office*, which just so happened to be playing "Dinner Party," my favorite episode, and I let it drown out the sounds of the hospital while I drifted off to sleep.

The evening was relatively uneventful other than being woken up every few hours to have my blood drawn. Everyone was so insistent that I get rest, yet this place was not exactly conducive to those efforts. I spent half the night sleeping, half the night staring at the clock, waiting for time to pass after being woken for labs in a cycle that continued throughout the night. Eventually, dawn would break, the new day would begin, and I set my sights on going home.

A new nurse entered my room with morning greetings and a menu in hand. "Would you like anything for breakfast?" she inquired.

It'd been over twenty-four hours since I'd eaten anything, so yes, breakfast sounded wonderful. She handed me the menu to look over while she wrote my goals on the board for the day.

Goal 1: Get up (move to the chair)
Goal 2: Get moving
Goal 3: Get discharged

After she finished writing the third, she enthusiastically suggested, "Let's get started with number one. How about we move to that chair, and you can eat breakfast from there this morning?"

She made that sound a whole lot easier than I thought it would be, given that every time I'd tried to stand up the day before, I'd nearly passed out. But I knew it was the first step to getting better, so I reluctantly agreed.

She called another nurse into the room, and they each steadied an arm as I swung my legs over the bed, braced myself for the pain, and then stood up. The pain was still there, but it didn't take my breath away this time, and as I opened my eyes, I realized I was standing . . . on my own . . . and I wasn't going to pass out this time. The nurse cheered as she encouraged me to take a few steps, and we walked over to the chair.

"Look at you!" she said. "You've earned that breakfast this morning. Anything sound good?"

I looked back at the menu. A blueberry muffin was calling my name, but the oatmeal sounded good as well. I wondered how much it would cost to order both as I searched for the prices. *I'm in a hospital; I imagine they charge an arm and a leg for everything.* When I couldn't find the price on the menu, I asked the nurse.

"I don't know, I can't decide between a muffin and some oatmeal. But I can't find the prices. Do you know how much they cost?" I asked, confused.

"Cost?" She looked back at me, equally confused.

"Yeah, my wallet is over there in my jacket. Maybe you can help me grab it? But I don't know how much it costs," I clarified.

She laughed. "Oh no, you don't pay for them on your card. It's all part of the hospital bill for being inpatient. It doesn't matter what you order; insurance typically takes care of it, and it's all lumped together. So order anything you'd like."

Anything I'd like? I thought. With my stomach grumbling, I felt like a kid who'd just been let loose in a candy store as I scanned back over the menu.

"Okay, I guess I'll take the blueberry muffin and some oatmeal then," I said as I continued to stare at the menu.

"Anything else?" she asked promptly.

"Maybe some orange juice and . . . maybe a piece of wheat toast too . . . ?" I cautiously replied, feeling like I was asking for too much. But I figured I could eat the oatmeal and toast for breakfast and save the muffin to snack on throughout the day. It felt like cheating, but they did say *anything*.

She chuckled again. "You got it. I'll place the order, and it'll be up shortly."

As I waited for my feast to arrive, Dr. Shaaban stopped by as promised. As he walked through the door, it took me a moment to place him, as he looked more like a business-man headed to the office than a doctor. He was dressed in a white button-down shirt, complete with a subtle lined pattern and a freshly pressed collar peeking through underneath the black wool winter coat he wore on top. The goatee and attire reminded me of my dad, who used to often sport a similar look on business trips. I swear you could have copied and pasted Dr. Shaaban's look and attire from my dad's during a business trip to New York he'd taken me on.

I was on the service of another doctor, who had already been by for rounds, so Dr. Shaaban wasn't here to place any orders or evaluate me for discharge. He was simply checking in. He didn't stay long this time, but I appreciated him taking the time out of his day to stop by. The visit might have been brief, but the effort spoke volumes.

Timed nearly perfectly, he left just as breakfast arrived. I took a bite of the blueberry muffin first. Mmmm . . . breakfast cake; who doesn't love muffins? The crumbs fell from my mouth as I savored each bite. I would have devoured the entire thing if it weren't for the intrusive thoughts that began to appear, chastising me for eating cake for breakfast. My mind shifted back to the week I'd been diagnosed and all the well-meaning friends, family, and strangers who were insistent on reminding me that sugar feeds cancer and it'd be best if I could avoid it altogether now. Which, I'll be honest, sounded pretty miserable. If the cancer was going to take me anyways, shouldn't I be enjoying my favorite things, not depriving myself of them?

I'd spent most of my life on some form of diet. In the last year, I'd had a dramatic weight loss, losing over fifty pounds with the help of diet, exercise, and who knows, maybe a little bit of cancer. I was walking up to ten miles a day, meal prepping, and counting macros. I definitely valued a healthy lifestyle, but at the same time, I still wanted a doughnut on my deathbed, not broccoli.

I wish I could say I overcame those thoughts and didn't let them get the best of me, but I didn't. After a few bites of the muffin, I packed it back away and set it to the side as I moved on to the oatmeal. I stared at the bowl of mush, pushing it around with my spoon before taking a bite. It tasted like lukewarm, flavorless goop. I saw the side of brown sugar next to it; I was certain it would make it taste better. But still plagued by the guilt of adding sugar to anything, I refused to let myself have any. After choking down a few bites and trying to convince myself I liked it, I began to gag. Okay, that was enough of that. Maybe I wasn't so hungry after all.

— 11 —

Food is NOT the enemy.

I'VE STRUGGLED WITH my weight my entire life. The flawed mindset of equating health with being thin was ingrained from a young age, even if I never achieved it.

One of my first memories, at the age of six, was "trying to lose weight" with my cousin: we raced around the house and in and out of every room, trying to get our cardio in. We'd start by weighing ourselves in my parents' bathroom upstairs before jogging around the top floor, navigating around and hurtling over obstacles in my siblings' rooms, then sprinting downstairs to the main level. From there we'd jog down the hall, into the bathroom, and tap our foot inside the door to my dad's office, which was strictly off limits-for our route, so we'd giggle about our rebellious rule break as we doubled back for laps around the TV room and kitchen and made three passes around the table before slowing our pace and "speed-walking" our way through the living room. Since it was full of nice furniture and fragile knickknacks, even on non-make-believe 5k route days there was a strict no-running policy. This was our cooldown before we'd head for our final leg of the race, down the stairs to the basement for our final lap before booking it back up both sets of stairs to recheck our weight to validate our progress.

Panting and out of breath, I stepped on the scale first: 48.8 pounds. *Dang it, it hasn't budged.* I felt a wave of disappointment rush over me as my cousin stepped on the scale: 41.2 lbs. While hers hadn't budged either, I was jealous she weighed less than I did. She was a year younger than me, but I'd often been compared to her in ways that even six-year-old me knew was referencing my weight. So when she said, "Let's go again," I tagged right along, hoping maybe another lap or two would do it. But much to my dismay, those extra laps didn't move the scale and instead only added to the complex I was already building.

As a kid, I was always the chubby one in class, with a few extra rolls around my waist. My parents divorced when I was two, and visits with whichever parent my brother and I weren't living with at the time always revolved around food; picking out our favorite snacks at the grocery store for weekend visits, Dairy Queen ice cream trips, and weekly dinner out as a family led to me equate food with love and comfort. These moments were always unrestricted and we were encouraged to enjoy ourselves, but outside those designated time slots, it was time to diet—something I began before the age of ten and carried with me in one form or another through adulthood.

However, no matter how much dieting and restricting myself I'd do, I was unable to get down to what I envisioned as an ideal body weight at the time. Which I believe largely had to do with the motives behind the efforts. It was never about my health; it was about my image. It was always to live up to a standard someone else had set that I internalized and adopted. Movies, magazines, boyfriends, and passing comments constantly shaped my image of what beauty looked like and served as reminders that it didn't look like me.

I envied my friends who could eat anything they wanted without gaining weight, and I often fantasized about all the foods I'd eat if I never had to worry about my size. In high school, I'd watch thinspiration videos online and envied the bodies of women with eating disorders, until I myself developed one of my own—but even that I was miserable at. I tried to starve myself in an effort to achieve the same results. However, that lasted all of a day before I gave in to my grumbling stomach and altered my tactics. Since I didn't have the willpower to starve myself, I started bingeing and purging instead. It never led to weight loss but usually held my weight steady for whatever phase of life I introduced it to, which would end up spanning a full decade. I purged heavily in my teens, but I never considered it a problem into adulthood, as I figured it was only a problem if you couldn't stop. I could stop, and I had done so several times to prove to myself that I could.

I treated it like a bridge, getting me from one diet to another, instead of like the eating disorder it was. It wasn't until my first health scare and the first trip to the ER in October 2019 that I truly woke up to my health and the cycle finally stopped. After that visit led to what felt like an endless pursuit of unexplained symptoms, I became discouraged. I knew something was wrong, but everyone kept telling me it was anxiety, and I didn't know what else to do. The medications they had prescribed me weren't working, and I couldn't get anyone to take me seriously, so I began taking matters into my own hands. It took a slap in the face via a health scare for me to recognize that my relationship with food shouldn't be about maintaining my image or body; it was about maintaining my health, something far more valuable than a flat stomach.

About six months before I met Brian, I was at my heaviest, 180 pounds on a short five-foot-one frame. I was no longer just overweight, according to the BMI index; I was classified as obese. Which, no matter how flawed a system it might be, made me feel terrible. I felt like I didn't have an excuse for letting my health slip, since my boyfriend at the time literally owned a gym. But I'd prioritized learning to code over sleep, eating a balanced diet, and exercise; I was living on fast food and snacks to power me through my evenings coding while he trained at the gym. We fought constantly over my weight and my perceived laziness, which only made me more resentful of working out. I was working full-time while building an app and teaching myself to code in the evenings. Every day, I'd work eight to ten hours at my day job, then program all night until four AM, leaving no time for friends or anything outside our relationship. When our multi-year relationship finally and abruptly crumbled during this period, the weight finally started to fall off, but this time it was a product of starvation and depression, not effort.

So when I met Brian, I had already lost a few pounds, but I was still embarrassed by my size—something that led to me delaying and pushing out our first meeting every time he asked to meet up because I was afraid he wouldn't be interested if he had a more complete picture of what I looked like. Thankfully, that wasn't the case and he loved me just as I was, but that didn't stop me from picking back up my bingeing and purging once being surrounded by a happy relationship led to a few pounds creeping back onto the scale. These behaviors aren't something I'm proud of and certainly not something I've ever openly shared. This book is the first time even Brian heard the full extent of the disorder I silently carried into our relationship. However, I choose to share it, because I think it's important to learn from our mistakes, and I hope that by sharing, not hiding behind my own, I can help empower others to choose different paths and feel a little less alone.

Opening up about my past struggles with an eating disorder isn't easy to do; however, it's important, not only because it aids in understanding my relationship with food and the insecurities I carried into my battle with cancer but also because it highlights a bigger problem that I wished I'd realized before it slapped me in the face. Our relationship with food shouldn't be about flat stomachs and earning the love and approval of those around us. Food is fuel for our health and our lives. Food should be balanced, and we should aim to make healthy choices, but at the end of the day, food is essential to life and is *not* the enemy. Which is something I didn't learn for myself until I began struggling with my health and food and exercise were the only levers I had left to pull.

After the ER visit, I decided to start working on my diet and well-being, this time not to live up to some beauty standard set before me but in an effort to preserve my health. Every time my heart rate went through the roof, it felt like my body was working overtime, even for the simplest of tasks. So I figured, maybe if I lost some weight, it wouldn't have to work so hard to pump blood around, and surely if nothing else, it couldn't hurt, right? So I revised my diet and began working out five times a week.

This time, I became much more disciplined about my diet. Brian and I stopped eating fast food, as I found it difficult to stay within the sodium limits I'd set for myself in hopes of it lowering my blood pressure. I also stopped drinking any alcohol or caffeine, which meant I was forced to cut out my daily trips to the gas station for an energy drink and a snack that I'd grown accustomed to. It was difficult to change my habits, but each time I was tempted to sway from my goals, my growing health issues loomed overhead as a reminder that maybe that cookie wasn't worth it.

My heart rate and blood pressure were still high, and even a walk around the block would often elevate it to 170/115 and leave my heart rate pinned at 165 bpm. So I took it slow and set small goals for myself. I didn't care how fast I walked, and I wasn't going to pressure myself to run; I simply needed to walk a quarter mile each day. That's it: a quarter mile and I could call it a success. Once I got that down, week by week, I graduated my distance to a half mile, a mile, then two miles by the end of 2019. Slowly, it wasn't just my body that was changing; I noticed my relationship with exercise had changed too.

Since I no longer had any illusions about running a marathon or competing for time, exercise wasn't a burden or a reminder of my failure if I couldn't keep up. Instead, it became therapeutic for me. It was a reminder of all my body could do instead of everything it couldn't. Sure, I couldn't run around the block, but a month before, I hadn't been able to walk around it, and now I was rounding my second loop. That was an achievement worth celebrating. Taking away all the external motivators allowed these daily escapes to become therapeutic adventures I looked forward to. It was time to be alone and think, time to observe and appreciate my surroundings and time to reflect.

These efforts paid off, and by the end of the year I was ten pounds down and had momentum to carry into the new year. So after COVID hit and shut the world down, I channeled all the uncertainty and anxiety into morning and evening walks, eventually working my way up to six to ten miles a day. I continued to improve my diet during this time and ultimately would lose fifty pounds in total by October 2020, just in time for my and Brian's wedding. I was proud of this progress, and while I looked better as well, more than anything, it changed my mind-set toward food and exercise.

I wish I could say that revising my diet rid me of all the symptoms I was feeling or that it cured the cancer. This isn't that kind of book; the fact that I'm even writing this book is proof that diet alone wasn't enough to slay Newman, the grapefruit-sized freeloader raging a war on my body. However, what it did teach me was how to have a better relationship with food, one that had been missing most of my life. One built on health, not image, where food is fuel and is meant to enhance your life, not deprive you of it. Sure, I had phases where I cut out fat, I cut out sugar, I cut out gluten, or I tried various elimination diets. However, this time they were part of a quest to learn more about my body, not an effort to deprive it of anything. When I tried each of these diets, it wasn't to lose an extra ten pounds, it was in exploration of what was causing me to feel so terrible. It was an experiment on myself that would allow me to become more attuned to my body. It helped me identify the very specific foods and scenarios that would trigger the severe abdominal cramps I was getting, and it allowed me to hone in on the bulge in my upper right abdomen that I likely wouldn't have noticed had I still been fifty pounds heavier.

I never want to go back to having a broken relationship with food and my body, but I'd be lying to you if I said being diagnosed didn't challenge those newly formed values. I didn't make it twenty-four hours into announcing my diagnosis before I had well-meaning messages filling my in-box with recommendations to immediately stop eating any and all forms of sugar, some of them without even a condolence sprinkled on top—and it really messed with my head. I already wasn't eating much in the days that followed the diagnosis. Food is a representation of love and comfort to me, but depression and lack of appetite are the other end of the spectrum. I was dropping weight quickly, and Brian began to notice.

"You have to eat," he'd beg me, offering to make all my favorite foods to get me to eat anything.

But I couldn't. Not only was I not hungry, but as I stared into the cabinet, it was as if there were now giant red warning labels strewed across every item I reached for. *I can't have a sandwich because the bread has gluten, which Cyndi says turns to sugar and is just as bad as a Snickers, but don't go for that banana either, because it'll spike your insulin. Joanne says no lunch meat because it's too processed and causes cancer. Dave recommends no meat at all because it's all carcinogenic. Sarah has it out for eggs because they raise your cholesterol, but Chad says cholesterol is a friend, not a foe: "Go ahead, fry that bacon; keto cures cancer," he insists.* There were contradictions everywhere I looked, but the one thing everyone seemed to agree on was that sugar was the devil. So I'd better toss the ketchup, packed with two grams of added sugar, *and don't even think about dessert.*

I knew better than to believe them all, but what if I was wrong? Would Dave stand at the pulpit at my funeral one day and read from his eulogy titled "Keto: the Murderer of Cows and Katie"? I mean, if I'd blatantly ignored his advice, could I really blame him? Which touches on the very core of the issue that had moved beyond the food itself. Inadvertently, all these suggestions had kicked me back down to the bottom of the hole I'd worked so diligently to dig myself out from, and I found myself making decisions not of my own free will but based on others' expectations of me. Which was fueled by both a fear of being wrong and a fear of becoming a disappointment to whoever had a recommendation I didn't follow in a time where I so desperately needed and craved their support. So rather than disappoint anyone, I'd open the cabinet doors, sit cross-legged on the floor staring into them, and sob. It was easier to not make a decision at all than to risk making the wrong one.

By the time my first appointment rolled around, I was losing weight quickly and knew it was becoming a problem. So I broached the topic with my oncologist, asking him if there were any modifications to my diet I'd need to implement. I was too embarrassed to ask him about sugar directly, knowing how controversial that topic might be, but since he'd clearly had that conversation many times before, he knew exactly what I was getting at. He recommended I eat a healthy balanced diet but said I didn't need to restrict myself and that I should be aiming to maintain my weight, not lose anything further—so if all that sounded good was a hamburger, then eat the hamburger. It was better to eat something than nothing at all. He explained that cancer will feed on anything, so even if I cut out all sugar or if I stopped eating entirely, my tumor would mutate to find other sources to fuel its growth. So everything in moderation and sugar isn't the enemy. His only ask was that

I stop taking any supplements like turmeric, which could have an effect on the effectiveness of immunotherapy if I went on treatment; it was best to avoid supplements and stick to getting my nutrition directly from food sources instead.

While these recommendations didn't get rid of the intrusive thoughts or the warning labels I saw on everything, it did give me the permission to ignore them. Which I needed more than anything—something I could point to as my reasoning for not following someone's recommendation, so I didn't have to be afraid of letting them down worried that the alternative would result in me losing their support. After that appointment, I'd still struggle to eat and the thoughts and recommendations still followed me around, preventing me from indulging in some of my favorite foods like the decadent blueberry muffin, the star of my hospital room breakfast feast. But the guilt of disappointing my loved one was gone, which finally broke my fast and allowed me to begin eating again.

— 12 —

*So as long as I'm still writing the story, this isn't how my
story ends, and now we fight.*
—Instagram post, January 20, 2021

AFTER A RATHER dramatic day, thankfully, the rest of my
hospital stay was largely uneventful. Within twenty-four
hours, although I was still in a fair amount of pain, I could get
up on my own and shuffle back and forth between the bed and
the chair. The improvement was noticeable.

With the progress I'd made, I was now set to be discharged.
As I finished lunch, I stared at the clock, counting down the
minutes until Brian arrived. I'd just married this man so we
could spend every night for the rest of our lives together. I'd
never anticipated I'd be giving one night up so soon, and quite
frankly, it was miserable. I was in no rush to do it again anytime soon. Before I knew it, I saw him walk through the door
and felt a crinkly-eyed smile spread across my face, which he
returned as he made his way over.

"I wish I could give you the biggest hug right now," I
expressed as I tightly squeezed his hand.

He chuckled. "Me too. I missed you!" He leaned down to
gently kiss my forehead as he began scanning the room. "The
pets did too, so let's get you home." He placed a beanie on my
head and grabbed my coat from the windowsill.

Still in a bit of disbelief about all that had transpired over the last day, I must have told him I loved him a hundred times on the way home as I opened up about how scared I'd been. He reciprocated and we both teared up. That experience gave us both a newfound appreciation of just how fragile life was, and we didn't leave each other's side for days afterward.

I was still in a decent amount of pain as we arrived back home, but the doctors had encouraged me to walk to help the healing process. So Brian would help me up every few hours, and we'd pace up and down the hallway together. I'd slowly put one foot in front of the other until I reached a thousand steps, then it was back to the couch, where I'd lounge and watch *Schitt's Creek* to pass the time until our next hallway adventure.

Before the biopsy, I'd been taking daily walks to clear my mind and help me cope. They were the one part of my life left unchanged since my diagnosis. I might no longer be the same, but the mile block of houses I weaved my way through and made laps around every day was. Every day, I'd been bundling myself up in a winter coat, two pairs of gloves, a scarf, and the warmest winter boots I could find before trekking across the neighborhood through the snow.

I'd start with a loop around the basketball courts and then make my way down to the main road, where I'd follow the sidewalk for several blocks. I didn't know the name of a single street on the block, but I could tell you a story about every dog. The first one I passed was a loud, aggressive dog that belonged to a duplex at the end of the street. He'd snarl and bark incessantly at me from the other side of the fence anytime I dared to walk on his side of the sidewalk. It didn't deter my longing to be his friend, but I found the BEWARE OF DOG sign posted on the gate fitting.

A few doors down from him were three Great Danes that in the summer I'd often see roaming the yard with their owners while they gardened. I always hoped they'd be out front so I could sneak a quick pet over the fence as I walked by.

I craved these walks while I was recovering, and I struggled to keep myself occupied without them. So by day three, when Brian offered to try a walk with me outside, I couldn't shuffle to my shoes fast enough. I typically took these walks alone—they were my time to think and reset—but I knew it probably wasn't wise for me to go on my own yet, and I looked forward to his company.

Walking might be one of my favorite pastimes, but it wasn't one of Brian's. A year ago, on a trip to Austin, I'd convinced him to go on a walk with me in uncomfortable shoes. I'd promised it would be short, maybe a mile or two at most. But by the time we'd finished, it'd morphed into five. He and his blisters never forgave me, and from that day forward, he tended to opt out of my casual "quick walk" invites. If he was the one offering this time, I knew I'd better strike while the iron was hot. Plus, due to the pain, I'd be unlikely to make it one mile, let alone five; surely he'd be safe.

We settled on a shorter loop, just around our immediate neighborhood, for this first outing, and as we walked hand in hand, I beamed with excitement. I told him stories about each of the dogs we passed along the way and which ones were my favorite. As I narrated our walk with childlike excitement, he looked over at me with a soft smile full of love. He might be one of the least outwardly expressive people I'd known, but he always found my excitement and curiosity rather endearing. I knew that look well. "I love seeing how happy these walks make you," he said. "Let's plan on this every day."

I whipped my head around. "Wait, what? Every day. Like willingly? You want to go on a walk every day?" I replied in disbelief.

He laughed. "I do. These walks make you happy, and I love seeing you happy." His tone quieted as I heard the emotion slip into his voice. "I want to spend as much time as I can with you, doing things that make you happy."

I stopped in my tracks. *Why'd he have to throw that line in there?* Life felt so much more fragile these days, since we were unsure of how much time we'd have together. We teared up as the weight of the statement hit us both. "A walk every day. You're going to regret that," I playfully tossed back with a smile in an attempt to stop both of us from becoming a puddle of tears.

He chuckled and said "Probably" as we continued on.

It didn't take long before those half-mile walks around the neighborhood graduated to one mile, then two. Every day I got a little stronger, the pain faded a little more, and I was left in true amazement at the resilience of the human body. I'd gone from being bedbound, unable to move without excruciating pain, to again walking laps around the neighborhood only a week later with nothing more than a dull ache from the bruises left behind. For days afterward, I'd catch myself breathing in and filling my lungs with the crisp winter air until reaching capacity, then taking a slow release to watch the crystals form on my breath as it all played out in reverse. I was left with an immense appreciation for the beauty in such a simple yet vital action I'd taken for granted a million times before, along with astonishment that it wasn't a medical intervention that had restored this ability over the past few days; it was healing my body had done on its own, simply given nothing but time.

The week between the biopsy and the results was filled with anxious waiting, but it was also filled with an unbelievable amount of gratitude I'd never felt before. An appreciation for all I'd previously taken for granted and the overwhelming love and support I felt from others as they rallied around me frequently brought me to tears.

Over the years, I'd built up a narrative in my head that I was a burden on everyone and too awkward, shy, and reserved to belong. I wasn't into surface-level conversations and struggled to speak up or connect in groups. Unable to relate to those around me, I was the wet blanket in every room, and I knew it. I'd often sit on the periphery, turning down every request to join in the fun while simultaneously beating myself up for not participating. It was like there was this invisible wall between me and any group I found myself in, and no matter how hard I tried, I couldn't seem to break through it. Eventually, I stopped trying altogether, and as much as it pained me to distance myself from those I loved, I figured they'd all be a lot better off and have a lot more fun if I never showed up. I began turning down invites, stopped attending family parties, and avoided any group gatherings, convinced I was doing everyone a favor.

So when my diagnosis came and a sea of family and friends came running to my aid, dropping off care packages and sending along words of encouragement, that narrative slowly began to crack. One particular instance that began to shift my perspective was when, in the days following my biopsy, my family dropped off a "box of sunshine"—a large cardboard box lined with yellow duct tape and filled with notes, balloons, snacks, and just about anything yellow that could be stuffed inside. As I opened it, I smiled and laughed before the river of tears began tracing their way down my face as I read the messages from my siblings, parents, nieces, and nephews that had even Brian tearing up. As I sorted through the box, it was filled with so much care and love that it made me feel incredibly grateful for my family. Unable to visit family and friends in the middle of the pandemic because I couldn't afford to have appointments rescheduled by a minimum of three weeks due to getting sick, these little gestures were one of our only forms of connection with loved ones, and they meant the world. But as I glanced back at each of the notes, I muttered softly under my breath, "This was so thoughtful. I don't deserve this."

Most people who know me well know how deeply I care for others, even strangers. When I see others hurt, I hurt, and I feel it to my core. I wear my heart on my sleeve and often actively seek out ways to help others. But I've always been terrible at being on the receiving end of that, often being far too stubborn for my own good. At the time, I was really struggling with admitting I was having a hard time or needed help, not wanting to inconvenience anyone.

I'd spent most of my adult life convincing myself that everyone in my life simply tolerated my presence and didn't actually like me. I might have been an introvert, but I often surrounded myself with extroverts, so I always felt like the plus-one, the required tagalong of the person whose company everyone really wanted. This left me feeling awkward anytime I found myself attending events alone or trying to make small talk with people I figured didn't actually want me around.

As I stared back at the notes in the box and looked at the cards, cookies, and other goodies that had arrived for Brian and me over the past few weeks, I felt truly humbled. I'd been trying to be more open and vulnerable since my diagnosis, sharing openly the good and the bad through social media, trying to be authentic and real. The rawness of this moment reminded me that being vulnerable wasn't just a matter of being open about the physical challenges and unknowns ahead but also about revealing the new emotional discovery and journey that came in tow. After pulling out and setting aside all the notes and cards I'd received, I made a post on social media that served as both my struggling and gratitude post for the day, opening up about these feelings, and I left the box front and center in the middle of our living room for over a week, trying to remind myself to stay positive in the dark days that followed.

After recovering from the biopsy, I was so grateful to be feeling well that I did a decent job of distracting myself from the anxiety and uncertainty of awaiting the results. Maybe even a little too well, as I quickly became tied up in the idea that the liver biopsy would come back benign. Anytime I'd let my mind wander or my eyes would fill with tears, I'd begin pacing around the house singing, "It's benign [*clap, clap*], everything's fine [*clap, clap*]; it's benign [*clap, clap*], everything's fine [*clap, clap*]" ad nauseam—a strange coping mechanism I'd picked up in an effort to keep myself from breaking down. Which backfired as the hopes I'd built up came crashing down with one phone call that changed everything.

I'd been pacing back and forth across the house to pass the time and keep myself from going stir-crazy when my phone began vibrating. I watched a number with an area code that matched the cancer center's flash across my screen. My stomach dropped. *Is this the call?* I took a deep breath and answered, trying to mask the nerves.

"This is Katie," I answered as confidently as I could.

"Hi, Katie, this is Dr. Swami." A quiet, calm voice came through from the other end of the line.

"Oh, hi, Dr. Swami. I didn't think you'd still be working," I replied, glancing back to the time on my phone as the nerves turned in my stomach. *Seven thirty PM. Why is he calling so late?*

"We just got your biopsy results back, and I wanted to give you a call tonight," he said, his voice both steady and heavy as he began to break the news. "Both the liver and the kidney biopsy have come back as an oncocytic renal neoplasm, which is quite rare," he informed me.

The gears in my head began turning as I tried to process the news. *Oncocytic—does that mean oncocytoma? That would be good news, right? Oncocytomas are benign; we wanted this to be an oncocytoma. Why did his voice sound so somber?* "So does that mean it's an oncocytoma?" I timidly replied, confused and certain I was mispronouncing my new diagnosis.

"Well, kind of, but this is different. The pathologist said it looks like an oncocytoma, but so does the liver lesion, which doesn't happen for oncocytomas. So they're calling it an oncocytic renal neoplasm instead," he clarified.

I felt the tears welling up behind my eyes. "Does that mean it's cancer?" I asked, my voice breaking with emotion.

There was a brief pause on the other end of the line; this news felt equally difficult for him to break. "It is. Since the liver tissue matches the kidney, it means the tumor has spread and metastasized, making this stage four kidney cancer."

Before he finished, the tears gave way, and I instantly crumbled to the floor. I'd spent all week praying for this to be an oncocytoma, praying it'd be benign. *How can it be cancer? Why is it cancer? I'm too young for cancer*... My thoughts spiraled as I tried to fumble out a response, but more tears were the only thing that came out.

I could hear the empathy in his voice as he continued, trying to provide both reassurance and to give me time to process. "I'm sure you have lots of questions. We'll answer everything we can. I've added you to the schedule on Friday, and we'll talk more about it then, including any next steps, okay?"

"Okay," I whispered softly as I tried to catch my breath. "Thank you for calling. I know it's late . . ." My voice trailed off as I tried to muffle my crying. But I wanted him to know how much I appreciated the call.

"Of course. I wanted to make sure to get you the results tonight. Think about your questions, and we'll see you in two days, okay?"

"Okay . . . ," I replied one final time before hanging up the phone.

I curled up into a ball as I dropped the phone to my side and tears flowed down my face. Brian made his way across the room, and I soon felt his warm embrace completely engulf me as he pulled me in close, comforting me while he patiently waited for the update.

"It's cancer!" I declared between muffled sobs into his chest.

I felt his arms tense up, and he let out a deep, concerned exhale as he pulled me in closer. "Did they say what kind?"

"Oncotyomic, onco-cytick . . . onco . . . I don't know how to say it, onco something. But it's cancer," I stammered out, trailing off in pain and disbelief.

"Oncocytoma? I thought that one wasn't cancer," he replied, trying to comfort me.

"That's what I thought too. But he said no, it's cancer, because it's in my liver too. They're the same, and it's stage four cancer," I said as my voice gave way and I broke back into uncontrollable sobs.

I updated him on the rest of the call—that I'd have an appointment on Friday and that we'd have more time to ask questions—as he held and comforted me on the stairs until the tears slowed and we began discussing next steps.

"Do we tell family?" I asked, staring down at the floor, knowing the pain this news would cause them too.

"Only if you want to. Whatever you're comfortable with," Brian insisted as he wiped a tear from my eye and gently kissed my forehead.

"I think I just want to rip off the Band-Aid. I don't know if I can handle questions right now, so I think I may just post," I replied.

"I think that's fine. Whatever you want to do. You don't need to tell anyone right now if you don't want to either. It's okay. Whatever you think is best."

Brian always knew the right thing to say in these moments. He gave me an endless amount of unwavering support to empower me to make the best decisions for myself. But I also secretly wished he could be making these decisions for me or that he had stronger opinions I could hide behind, so I didn't have to be the one to make the call.

I knew so many others were pulling for me, all praying and hoping the results would be benign just like we had been. While I knew I didn't have the strength to field questions that I myself didn't even know the answers to yet, I had many loved ones waiting on pins and needles, and they deserved to know too. So I drafted a raw post on Facebook and Instagram with the title Results are in and tonight I don't want to be strong to bring everyone up to speed. It concluded with a message of hope that read:

> I'm scared, I'm terrified, and I'm devastated. But I'm going to push on and I'm going to fight. We're going to search wherever we can to find someone who knows anything about this type of cancer and I'm going to fight Newman and all his little friends with everything I've got.
>
> There have been several moments in my life that I never thought I'd be strong enough to face and a couple I've felt lucky to make it through alive.
>
> "If you can't beat fear, do it scared."
>
> Tonight I'm not beating the fear; it's raw, it's new and that's just what comes with the territory. But I'm going to push forward and fight this. I have a husband beside me, friends and family behind me and a whole life ahead of me I still want to live. So as long as I'm still writing the story, this isn't how my story ends, and now we fight.
>
> But tonight, tonight we just cry.

Returning to this post years afterward still gives me chills. I knew my cancer was rare, but I didn't know it was single-digits rare at the time of posting or the near impossibility of just about everything I wrote. I was broken and shattered but also filled with a blind optimism paired with a relentless drive and determination to change my circumstances. This was my first stand, my declaration that I wasn't going down without a fight and a proclamation that as long as I'm still writing the story, this isn't how my story ends.

— 13 —

We're going to search wherever we can to find someone who knows anything about this type of cancer and I'm going to fight Newman and all his little friends with everything I've got.
—Instagram post, January 20, 2021

BRIAN AND I had prepared for the scenario where we received bad news, but it didn't make the news itself any easier once it came. And now we were left with myriad decisions to make. It felt like an impossible task while juggling intense emotions, but we knew we didn't have time to waste.

One of the very first things I did after receiving my biopsy results was to look up as much information as I could on rare kidney cancers, breaking all of my "stay-off-Google" rules. But with a new piece of the puzzle, it felt like I was in a race against time to fill in as much of the picture as I could before my appointment Friday. I still might not have the expertise to filter search results or apply context to what I was finding, but my oncologist did. So I compiled a list of questions about things I didn't understand that I could bring him.

I typed in a search for "Rare Kidney Cancers" and hit enter. One of the first results was a webinar recorded just a few days ago. I thought of Daniel's advice: "Don't Google; you'll find a bunch of old stats and trials." *It was just posted, so those rules don't apply, right?* I told myself as I clicked on the link.

The video opened to a webinar from the Judy Nicholson Foundation, hosting Dr. Pavlos Msaouel, from one of the top-rated cancer centers in the world, MD Anderson in Houston, Texas, discussing rare kidney cancers. Perfect, exactly what I was looking for. I pressed play and let the video play out. It started with a high-level overview of kidney cancer and dove into the treatments, then the subtypes of kidney cancer, all of which respond differently to treatment. The information was well presented and far easier to grasp than any content about rare kidney cancer I'd encountered before. For the first time, I actually felt like I was understanding something and that it wasn't all going over my head. Dr. Msaouel emphasized the importance of knowing the subtype, and he discussed each type in detail and how they might differ in response to treatment on a slide with big bold lettering: "Kidney Cancer is Not A Singular Entity."

The slide had images with tiny pink circles and dots at the top of each column, displaying the histology, or the microscopic appearance, of each subtype, followed by the incidence rate, prognosis, and therapeutic targets of each. I saw "chromophobe" listed at the top of one column, a type still listed in my differential diagnosis in my pathology report. The prognosis was "very good." I blinked to make sure I'd read that correctly as I felt the hope begin rising. *Maybe I do have chromophobe*, I thought to myself. I clung tightly to that hope until I heard the words "but sometimes that may not be the case, which is why it's important to look at each patient as an individual." My stomach dropped again. The more I learned, the more I was absolutely fascinated by the nuance while simultaneously nauseated by everything I heard, trying to stomach and interpret prognosis estimations and determine how they might fit the disease currently raging a war inside me.

When I asked Dr. Swami about chromophobe RCC and if he had seen any patients with it, I received vague answers—a lot of "we have seen" and "we have treated" remarks that led me to believe he himself hadn't seen many cases. Both that and a haunting comment from my first appointment replayed in my mind: "Chromophobe usually doesn't spread to different parts of the body, but if it spreads, it's bad, because it doesn't respond to most things." I collected these reflections along with the newly acquired information I'd learned from the video, and I brought this context with me into my appointment with Dr. Swami to discuss the biopsy results. When he recommended immunotherapy as my front-line treatment, since it was what had worked best in clear cell renal cell carcinoma, the most common type of kidney cancer, I remembered the words in the video I'd watched a few days prior, highlighting the importance and differences between subtypes, including the limited responses in chromophobe kidney cancer to immunotherapy.

I knew Dr. Swami was extremely intelligent; he was empathetic and he was an incredible listener. It was clear he knew his stuff, but also that chromophobe kidney cancer wasn't his area of expertise. So when I asked if I could get a second opinion before starting treatment, he not only agreed but encouraged it, saying, "Of course, a second or a third, whatever you need." I was relieved to have his support, and Brian and I began the search. Dr. Swami wanted to get me started on treatment as soon as possible, which meant if we were going to get a second opinion at a hospital other than Huntsman, the time was now.

I didn't have a clue where to begin, and after an exhaustive search for "best hospitals for cancer," "best kidney cancer hospitals," and "best kidney cancer centers in the United States" resulted in little success, I decided to start with the center most commonly listed and the one the physician from the video I'd watched on rare cancers was from: MD Anderson Cancer Center. The next morning I sat cross-legged on the bed, puffy eyed, with a box of tissues next to me, and placed my first call to MD Anderson.

I didn't make it the first minute into the call before I broke down in tears, apologizing profusely to the woman on the other end of the line for my inability to hold it together. It was clear I wasn't the first person to have broken down on her. "Oh, honey, please don't apologize. This is hard stuff," she reassured me.

Sensing my urgency, she booked the earliest appointment available with the first free genitourinary oncologist (GU), a doctor who treats patients with prostate, kidney, bladder, and testicular cancer. I'd notified her that I had a very rare type of kidney cancer and wanted to be seen by someone who treated rare kidney cancers but was reassured all of their GU specialists could. Something at the time I didn't know I needed to push further.

The earliest they could get me in was February 2, about two weeks away, but I'd need to arrive three days prior so I could be tested for COVID and quarantined in the hotel until my appointment. Which meant we had a little over a week to book flights, a hotel, and transportation and to find pet care. While I was relieved to have one item checked off the list, I was overwhelmed by the other five I'd managed to add. Thankfully, Brian swooped in to take care of the rest as I lay in bed and sobbed.

I was overwhelmed, but I knew the decisions didn't stop there. We'd decided to go to MD Anderson for a second opinion, but we still needed to determine what that meant for our housing if we decided to switch my care. Through support groups and insight from family friends who'd gone to MD Anderson while living out of state, we knew we didn't have to live there to pursue treatment. We could feasibly still live in Utah, and I could fly in for treatment and scans. However, as I began budgeting out our cost, it became clear we couldn't cover treatment, travel, and our new mortgage. It was time to have the conversation I'd dreaded since the day I was diagnosed. It was time to talk about giving up the house.

We'd driven down every weekend for months to watch it come together and daydream about the life we'd build in it. Now that we were just over a month away from it being finished, giving up on it now didn't feel like we were just giving up on a house—it felt like giving up on our future. But with the uncertainty we both knew we'd be facing, the numbers just didn't add up. It was time to let go.

That night I didn't get an ounce of sleep. My life was crumbling right before my eyes, and there was nothing I could do to stop it. I felt hopeless. So I turned to the only group of people I imagined could understand: other patients in a stage four kidney cancer group online.

> I'm really struggling with the diagnosis tonight. I can't sleep, am really nauseous, and honestly really scared (haven't started treatment yet).
>
> Any tips for sleeping or learning to cope? I could also really use success stories from anyone who was diagnosed at stage 4.
>
> I have a very large, uncommon tumor that very rarely spreads but it's spread to my liver, in at least 6 spots, several large (~5 or 6 cm).
>
> They don't have a prognosis for me based on how rare my tumor is and told me they may have a better idea at my 3 month scans.
>
> Sorry to post here so much but you all have been so welcoming and comforting. And I just need a little help tonight.
>
> Any success stories or tips on how to manage sleep would be greatly appreciated.

The comment section was quickly filled with suggestions and inspiring stories of hope. Many shared their sleep remedies, what was working for them, and recommendations on things to ask my doctor about. Others offered up their success stories—like Meridith, who'd been on treatment for two years and was doing great, still gardening and spending time with grandkids. "Don't give up hope," she encouraged.

I met my friend Laura after I made this post. She shared her story, which was similar to mine: she too had been diagnosed at twenty-nine with a similar-sized tumor of a rare subtype in the ER. She'd undergone an intensive surgery, then found out the cancer had spread to her liver and a few other locations during follow-up scans. After a clinical trial, she was now off treatment with no evidence of disease. We had different types of kidney cancer and different amounts of disease, but I didn't need to know I'd have the same response; I just needed to know *someone* had had this kind of response, that it wasn't impossible and that there were others my age still alive. She was that someone, and we built a friendship over our commonalities in and outside of cancer on the foundation of hope.

I couldn't help but notice the support group's positivity, a theme I admired in the other posts on the page. I appreciated the support these wonderful strangers so generously offered, and I wondered how they were able to handle their diagnosis with such grace and positivity, given the gravity of our shared circumstances—a mind-set I so desperately wished I could acquire but couldn't seem to manage no matter how hard I tried.

Before the cancer was confirmed in my liver, it was easier to live in denial. I'd begun focusing on and appreciating all my body was capable of instead of all that my body couldn't do as I recovered from the biopsy. But now the negative intrusive thoughts and the feeling of impending doom resurfaced as if there were a heavy dark cloud looming overhead, following me everywhere I went. The past few days, I'd thought I'd been doing better mentally, but it felt as if I were right back to square one. It was clear this mental battle wasn't going to be a linear path.

Everyone kept telling me to be positive, not to give up hope, and that my mind-set would be just as important as the treatments in the coming days. Which sounded great in theory, but my biggest question was how—how exactly does one just become positive? I'd often sit quietly, with my eyes closed, and try to focus on the things I was grateful for.

Brian and our marriage were always at the top of the list. I'd focus on how grateful I was to have him in my life and by my side, flashing back to memories of our wedding day. However, those reflections would quickly be taken over by intrusive thoughts about the pain I'd cause him when I passed or wondering who he'd marry when I was gone and if my memory would be replaced. Any positivity I'd managed to muster up was immediately crushed by the cascading thoughts and tears that followed.

As I watched other patients continuing with their lives, I wondered if something was wrong with me. Was I not trying hard enough? How were they smiling and enjoying their time with family and friends while I was still struggling to get past the tears? As I spiraled, I was so desperate that my search history became littered with search strings looking for answers: "happy with cancer," "how to be happy with cancer," "cancer success stories," "how to keep living after a cancer diagnosis." I scoured YouTube, Google, and Instagram hashtags in hopes I'd find someone who'd traveled the path before me and who might have documented the secrets. But other than a couple hundred more "be positive" recommendations, I came up empty. Which only reaffirmed my desire to continue sharing my experience online. If I ever managed to find the elusive answer along the way, maybe my journey could act as someone else's how-to guide one day.

Trying to be conscious of the battle ahead and any surgeries I might have, Brian and I knew staying in the townhome wouldn't be a great option. It'd be easiest to live somewhere with a single level, with minimal stairs and a yard for Baxter. But it'd need to be something we could afford on one income in case I was unable to work. This soon became what felt like a near-impossible task as we spent several hours a day browsing through listings and inquiring about properties.

Apartments wouldn't be a great option, because most of them weren't pet friendly and the one or two that were only had units available on the third floor. We moved on to looking for houses, basement apartments, and single-level townhomes, where we encountered the same issues. The only pet-friendly units either didn't allow dogs, didn't allow cats, or were out of our budget. A tear silently slipped down my cheek as I clicked through listing after listing, feeling hopeless. Why did so many rentals in Utah have restrictions against pets?

Brian, browsing listings on his own, looked over and caught the tears in my eyes. "You okay?" he gently asked.

"I'm not finding anything. I'm worried we're not going to find anything," I replied, the hopelessness and frustration evident in my voice.

The next words to come from his mouth were words I'd never thought I'd hear him speak. "What about Texas?"

I shifted my eyes up toward him, confused. "What do you mean, what about Texas?" I asked.

"What if we look in Texas?"

I looked down and shook my head as if to clear my thoughts. I was sure I must have misheard him. "Wait, what? You want to look in Texas?" I asked in disbelief.

"I've been working remotely since COVID started, and they aren't asking people to come back to the office until at least July. I'll ask if I can move into a permanently remote position, or I'll have until July to find another job," he reassured me. "I know Texas and Austin make you happy. I want you to be happy," he said as I caught the glimmer of moisture welling up behind his eyes before he turned back to his computer. "I've been looking at listings, and from what I've seen so far, our dollar will go a lot further there. Almost everywhere I've looked is pet friendly."

He pulled up a listing, a ground-floor apartment with a small yard and modern finishes. "It doesn't have to be this one. This is just an example, but there are several like this. We could look in Houston or Austin, and either would put you closer to MD Anderson if we decide we like it there."

There was no doubt that Austin was my happy place. It'd become home for me, and I missed everything about it. But when we decided to build the house, I'd given up on the dream that we'd ever find our way back there, and I'd fully accepted it. "But Texas is hot, like really hot, and you hate the heat." I rebutted cautiously, trying not to get my hopes up, certain he must have offered up the suggestion without fully thinking it through.

He let out a subtle chuckle. "Yes, yes I do," he said. "But you hate the cold, which is just as important. I'm inside ninety-nine percent of the time; you're always out for walks. As long as you give me AC, I'm fine. I didn't just decide on this; it's something I've been thinking about a lot."

My eyes quickly began filling with tears of joy. "You're serious?" I confirmed one more time as I felt the smile spreading across my face.

He nodded his head slightly and laughed. "Yes, I'm serious. It's completely up to you, but that option is on the table."

I smiled and stared off into the distance for a minute, letting the news sink in.

"We're moving to Texas . . . ," I muttered quietly under my breath. I closed my eyes and pictured the warmth of the sun on my skin and heard the crunch of the gravel beneath my feet as I walked along my favorite path. "We're moving to Texas . . . ," I repeated a little louder, the excitement and smile growing on my face before I turned and looked at Brian. "We're moving to Texas!!!" My smile was as wide as the state itself. It turned up the corners of my eyes and forced out a tear from the puddle that had been collecting as I excitedly tapped him on the leg.

He began to laugh. "Wait a second. We're not moving yet." He'd have been kidding himself if he thought suggesting we could move back to Austin would elicit any other reaction from me. But I humored him as he halfheartedly tried to apply the brakes. "We don't even have a place yet, and you might not like MD Anderson . . . but if you do . . . it's an option," he said, with a playful smirk on his face that gave me full permission to continue daydreaming.

"Right," I said as I furrowed my brow and pretended to temper my excitement. "You're right. I might not even like MD Anderson . . . the number-one cancer center in the world. It's probably terrible." My tone was laced with sarcasm as I tried to force a frown.

"Exactly," he said, chuckling.

I looked back at my laptop as I swapped out the location from Salt Lake City to Austin in my search. "We're moving to Austin . . . ," I whispered under my breath, a subtle smile resurfacing.

He playfully rolled his eyes while sliding across the couch to join me. "You know . . . I know you love Austin and all, but you really could have found a less dramatic way back. You didn't *have* to get cancer," he teased as he placed his hand on my knee, squeezing three times, our universal sign for *I love you*.

"All part of my master plan," I replied between laughs. "Good thing I'm so good at planning," I added, making myself laugh now, knowing how much my lack of day-to-day planning drove him crazy. I'd always been super organized and ten steps ahead at work or in making long-term plans, but day-to-day I was far more spontaneous than he was. Last-minute adventures without a plan, cooking without a recipe, hanging pictures on gut feel—that was my jam. But him, not so much—that was a surefire way to stress him out.

"Oh god, I'd hate to see what you have planned next," he mocked back, with a mixture of amusement and fear.

— 14 —

MD Anderson sees an insane number of patients and my oncologist has never seen a patient with an oncocytoma that has metastasized (neither had my Dr. at Huntsman).
—Instagram post, February 2, 2021

WITH THE FULL support of our families, I began packing and preparing for the move to Texas so that if things went well at MD Anderson, we'd be ready to pick up and go. Or at least as ready as someone can be when planning and executing a move within a week, half of which we'd be out of town for. But focusing on the move was a good distraction. Working kept me occupied during the day, but any second I was left unoccupied with my thoughts outside of work, the emotions, fear, and uncertainty would creep in. So I began filling any downtime I had left with boxes, packing tape, and Styrofoam wrap to drown out the anxiety.

I'd moved a lot as a kid, a habit that I'd somehow managed to pick up and unintentionally take with me into adulthood. With over thirty moves behind me in my short lifetime so far, I was a true expert. Give me a room and I could tell you how many boxes it would fill and how long it would take to pack. I enjoyed the busywork of finding the right items, box sizes, and categories to break down a room into, so each box would be perfectly filled to the top without becoming too heavy to carry. By the end of the week, any item that wasn't still in use had been carefully packed away in its place. Boxes lined the walls to greet us on our return.

The morning of our flight, Brian's mom picked us up to take us to the airport. Even though Brian and I were married, I had interacted with his mom only a few times. We'd met for the first time at Thanksgiving 2019, after Brian and I had already moved in together, and we'd only gotten together a few times before COVID hit. We hadn't really had the chance to get to know each other well, and honestly, we still felt more like strangers than in-laws. I'd been crying all morning, so I cleared the makeup from under my eyes and tried to hold it together as I opened the door to the back seat. As I climbed in, I spotted the bottle of water and box of tissues Brian's mom had placed on the middle seat for me—a small gesture that meant the world to me. Regardless of the limited time we'd spent together, I knew this was her way of saying, *You're family, and we're here to support you.* I buckled in and grabbed a few tissues from the box to soak up the newly formed droplets behind my eyes, stashing a few in my pocket for later. I knew the emotions would likely be resurfacing all day.

When we got to the airport and checked in, Brian handed me my ticket. "I did something," he said as he tried to suppress a smile. "But don't be mad," he added.

"What did you do?" I looked down at the ticket and back up at him, confused.

"I upgraded us," he responded confidently.

"For more legroom?" I asked. Coming in at six foot one, Brian was nearly a foot taller than I. I wouldn't blame him if he'd upgraded for more space. Why had he told me not to get mad?

"No, to first class," he clarified, as his stoic expression cracked and a smirk began peeking through.

"Wait, what?" I asked as I glanced down at the ticket and back up at him. I'd never flown first class before; the prices were so astronomical I'd never even considered it. I must have heard him wrong.

"I knew how difficult today was going to be, and I wanted you to be comfortable. So I called and upgraded us to first class," he said as he saw my eyes refill once more and he pulled me in for a hug.

I wrapped my arms around him, and his jacket pressed against my cheek, muffling my reply. "But tickets are so expensive," I argued as I shifted my positioning, looking straight up and into his eyes. "I don't need it. It's too expensive. You really didn't need to do that," I argued once more. My diagnosis had already meant us giving up the house, and I worried the medical expenses would only continue to rack up from here. I felt guilty and worried about the financial drain I seemed to have become.

"I know you don't need it . . . but you deserve it," he replied. "Don't worry about how much it cost. No one is flying right now; it was actually pretty cheap. We won't do it every time, just this time. This is going to be a hard trip. I want you to be comfortable."

I turned my head and embraced him tightly as the tears collected in my mask. This man was beyond anything I could ask for in a partner. I couldn't have been more grateful for his love but found myself simultaneously bitter at the life circumstances trying to cut our love story short. All I wanted was more time with him; hopefully, MD Anderson could reset the clock.

Once we arrived, I didn't sleep a wink as I lay in bed, poking and prodding at my stomach, feeling around for Newman. It'd officially been one month since my diagnosis. I still wasn't on treatment, and my mind raced as I mentally measured the boundaries and edges of the tumor, searching for any signs or indications of growth. I didn't know when I'd be starting treatment after getting the second opinion, but I hoped it would be soon so I could stop worrying about the cancer growing unchecked and I could finally feel like we were doing something.

As morning rolled around, Brian and I both arose early and got a jump-start on work—something that I look back on now with a bit of sadness. That afternoon, I'd be sitting across the room from a stranger in a white coat inquiring about how much time I had left to live. Yet here I was, worried about how much PTO I'd taken and trying to conserve it for however much time I had left before the cancer took over. That day, I'd work for several hours in the morning, go for my appointment, then come back and work several more hours in the afternoon and into the evening to make up for the time I'd stepped away.

I'd always heard people talk about how they'd spend their final days if they found themselves with a limited time left to live. It was always some variation of quitting their jobs, traveling the world, and spending time with family and friends. I mean, in theory, that sounds like a pretty decent way to go out. However, when I was in that position myself, the days looked far less glamorous. Instead of jet-setting across the country, I was buffering thirty-minute windows to allow myself to break down after receiving life-altering news before pulling it back together and hopping on a Zoom call to finish out the day.

This sounds like I had a horrible employer, but that couldn't be further from the truth. Everyone at work was actively encouraging me to take time off, but up until this point in my life, work had been not only my escape but my entire identity. I didn't know how to function or fill the time without it. I was constantly worried about the work I'd leave behind for others to pick up if I wasn't around. It wasn't my boss or my coworkers guilting me into work; it was me who couldn't let go. I was too stubborn to take the time. In retrospect, while work was a nice distraction, I wish I hadn't pushed myself so hard during that time. There are far more important things in life than work.

But some lessons you can only learn the hard way . . . at least if you're a twenty-nine-year-old woman whose fatal flaw is being stubborn to a fault—a trait I'm not proud of and one that cancer would continually challenge me to reshape with time.

By midmorning, it was time to head over for my appointment. We had so much riding on it that my mind was racing and my heart was beating out of my chest. So as a distraction, I started making nervous small talk focusing on our surroundings instead. There was one city block between the hotel and the Mays clinic where my appointment would be, and as we rounded the corner, I tilted my head back and looked up toward the sky.

"Can you believe how many buildings there are here?" I said, the astonishment filling my voice as I began counting the buildings with MD ANDERSON displayed prominently on the side. "I swear, just this area alone is bigger than downtown Salt Lake."

"I wouldn't be surprised," he said as he too turned his gaze upward.

Our route took us along the edge of the Texas Medical Center, a medical complex that covers a 2.1-square-mile radius, the largest in the world. I was speechless as I took in its sheer size. The craziest part of it all was that it wasn't even a part of downtown Houston. It was solely the medical district, filled with some of the best hospitals, clinics, and labs and the best-ranked cancer center in the world. I felt a sense of comfort as we walked alongside the towering buildings. If I wasn't in good hands here, I didn't know where else I would be.

Unfortunately, that feeling was fleeting and my mind began to wander as the weight of that statement sank in. In place of comfort, anxiety reappeared. We were now at the top of the chain, seeing the best of the best. What would that mean if they didn't have answers for me either? Would that be the end of the line? I felt the tears welling up behind my eyes again as I shifted my focus back to our surroundings once more.

Buildings and hospitals covered every square inch around us, but as I looked up ahead, I noticed a small open green space tucked off to the side of a building we were approaching. It was beautifully landscaped, with pavilions, picnic tables, and benches scattered throughout. As we passed, I took note of a retaining wall made of steel wire and filled with tiny smooth rocks that looked out of place among the open rockscaping in the rest of the park.

"Look at those poor, caged rocks," I said to Brian, gesturing to the wall and clearly grasping at straws with more nervous small talk to fill the silence. "Do you think they ever get jealous of the free rocks over there?" I asked as I pointed toward a large patch of scattered rocks beneath a tree ahead.

"Possibly," he replied with an endearing laugh. "I don't think rocks have feelings, though," he rebutted with a smirk.

Unfazed, I continued, "I think they're sad. I mean, just look at them. They just have to sit there and stare at the free rocks all day long. I mean, I'd be jealous if I were them."

"You're right. They're probably jealous," he admitted, shaking his head and rolling his eyes with a smile.

"I know," I confirmed, confidently lifting my head and broadening my shoulders as if to gloat in his admission of my being right. "Poor rocks," I said, reaching for his hand and smirking, a silent *Thanks for playing along.* His hand met mine, and he squeezed three times as we stepped into the crosswalk on our final stretch to the Mays building a few hundred feet ahead.

Once we reached the entrance, Brian passed along words of encouragement as we parted ways at the door and I shuffled in behind the other patients arriving for their appointments. Just inside, we queued up behind a screener who handed everyone a mask and asked that we sanitize as we entered before ushering us into a longer line down the hall. This one had big red social-distancing squares stuck to the carpet, each spaced six feet apart to queue up and guide the line into a large room at the end of the hall. I took my place in line and snapped a picture to document the moment. I might never have grandkids to tell these stories to one day, but if I made it through this, this would surely be a pretty crazy experience to look back on or at least to tell Brian about later. Cancer in the middle of a pandemic—zero out of ten recommend.

I followed the line down the hall into a sizable banquet-sized room that continued to twist and turn until reaching the three-sided MD Anderson–branded ticket booths that lined the back of the room. I stood in front of the booth and checked in with the receptionist after a frazzled fumbling through my records in search of my medical record number, which I hadn't thought I'd need to have memorized. She verified my appointment, then ran through a series of screening questions before giving me the all clear. I checked in one more time with the clinic before finding a seat in the lobby.

The furniture reminded me more of a living room than a doctor's office. Comfortable lounge chairs sat around coffee tables, medical recliners were arranged near the windows for a view, and several fish tanks broke up the space. I grabbed one of the chairs around an empty coffee table, set down my giant accordion file of medical records, and pulled out a notebook and pen to run through my questions as if I were prepping for an interview. The nerves turned in my stomach.

I tried to keep focused on the paper as I felt the eyes of other patients in the lobby who'd followed me in as the heels of my boots thumped across the floor. I'd been advised by another patient to be sure to put my best foot forward at my first appointment. "Part of your prognosis is calculated based on how you look when you enter the room, so don't look like you're dying," they'd advised. So I'd come well dressed, my hair curled and sporting the new heeled boots I'd bought for Christmas. Later, I'd realize this advice was geared toward influencing the Karnofsky Performance Status (KPS), an index that gauges a patient's ability to continue normal daily-life activities and is used to evaluate a patient's overall well-being and assist in prognosis assessment. After learning about the KPS index later in my diagnosis and realizing that's where this advice might have been pointed, I can't say I passed along the same to others. It's important not to mask how you've been feeling. But I had to admit, changing out of my sweats for the first time in weeks felt nice.

As I sat in the lobby, I already felt like I didn't belong, but the eyes of other patients around me didn't help. None of us were allowed to bring family to our appointment, and I couldn't help but feel like they were trying to determine how I'd managed to skirt the rules, looking for the dad or grandfather I must be accompanying. Kidney cancer is most common in men over sixty-five, so as a twenty-nine-year-old and the only woman in the waiting room, there was no denying I stood out like a sore thumb.

I don't belong here, I thought to myself as my leg nervously bounced and my hands began to shake. The nerves were mounting. I tapped the heart icon on my watch to check my heart rate: 142 beats per minute. I took a deep breath and locked my eyes on the reading, trying to get it to come down before they called me back for vitals. 141 . . . 139 . . . 138 . . . 136 . . . I continued to focus on my breathing as a notification popped on the screen. It was a text from Brian.

He had sent me a picture of a rock and a little green bubble with one word in it. Freeeeedom, it read. A smile spread across my face. Looked like he'd freed one of those rocks that didn't have feelings on his way back to the hotel. Who says romance is dead? Feeling a tad smitten and a little less anxious, I welcomed the distraction as we messaged back and forth.

As I waited, I texted Brian the play-by-play of my appointment. First up was vitals, then I was called back into a room, where I'd meet with the medical assistant and nurse practitioner to run through my history before my oncologist finally entered the room.

As she entered, she carried herself with a gentle but confident nature that felt warm and welcoming. After our introductions, I asked if I could record the appointment just as I had at Huntsman, since my husband was unable to be there with me. Although she informed me we couldn't record, she encouraged me to call him instead, so he could still listen in and be a part of the appointment. So that's exactly what we did. I pulled out my phone and patched Brian in over Face-Time on his laptop. I held him next to me the entire appointment with the camera facing toward my oncologist so it was almost like he was there. It felt so unnatural and strange, but I was grateful to have him with me in any capacity I could.

The appointment went well, and although I was a little concerned that it didn't sound like the oncologist had seen many patients with rare kidney cancers or who were as young as me before, I was impressed by her intelligence and felt that I'd be in good hands in her care. She still didn't have the official results from my Huntsman biopsy, which they'd evaluate again at MD Anderson; that meant there were no treatment decisions to be made that day, but the next steps from here would be for me to get a more complete workup. She'd add in labs and a bone scan to check for spread to my bones before she took my case to the tumor board the following week so she could evaluate and discuss my treatment plan with her colleagues. We'd regroup for a follow-up after that.

I left the appointment nervous that it'd still be weeks until I started treatment and worried about how long it might take to get in for scans. But within ten minutes of leaving the room, I'd already received notifications scheduling my labs and a bone scan for later that day. The size and speed of this place was insane.

The next day, Brian and I drove out to the coast to talk through the decisions ahead. I wanted to see the ocean before we left, and long drives always brought me peace. However, that peace was relatively short-lived, as the results of my scan hit my chart halfway through the drive. I tried my best to ignore the buzzing and the little red notifications, but as each new one slid in, my willpower dwindled, and it wasn't long before I gave in. As I pulled up the results, I began scanning through each record. My labs were still relatively normal—my blood counts had normalized from all the biopsy drama and there were only a few numbers left still out of bounds—but most importantly, my bone scan had come back clear. I let out a sigh of relief as I read the results out loud to Brian. I'd still have a full-body CT in a couple weeks for restaging as I started treatment, but for now, it looked like it was my kidney and liver we were dealing with.

With the results out of the way, we began recounting and talking through the past few days. We were satisfied with how things had gone at MD Anderson, we liked my oncologist and how quickly everything moved, and we'd even managed to make a couple new friends in town, Marvin and Debbie, who'd reached out to me after I posted in the support group asking for stories of hope and tips on sleeping.

Marvin was first diagnosed in 2012, but they'd moved to Houston to go to MD Anderson after his cancer recurred in 2016. We'd chatted with him and his wife, Debbie, on the phone several times before we came down, and while we were in town, they'd come up to meet us for coffee at the hotel. We might not have known them for long, but they welcomed us like family. If we decided to move, even though we'd be in an unfamiliar city fifteen hundred miles from home, between them and my stepbrother, who lived just outside of Houston, we felt we had the beginnings of a support system. So arriving at the coast, we also arrived at our decision. As Brian and I walked along the boardwalk and watched the sunset, we solidified our plans. By the end of the week, Texas would be our new home.

— 15 —

I'm ready for this new chapter and our move tomorrow but goodbyes, boy are they hard.
—Instagram post, February 5, 2021

AFTER RETURNING TO Utah from MD Anderson, Brian and I had exactly seventy-two hours until the movers arrived. In that time we'd need to finish packing up the house and say our goodbyes to loved ones. Luckily, our friends and family offered tons of help. My mom stopped by to run loads out to donation centers. Brian's dad brought dinner and helped us declutter. A friend dropped off snacks, a travel blanket, and road trip essentials for the car ride, and both my family and Brian's offered to tag-team our move out checklist and take on any final cleaning once we were out. I've always hated asking for or admitting I need help, but it meant the world to see the way our families and friends rallied around us. We definitely wouldn't have made it out of there in time without them.

As we wrapped up our packing, I had one last emotional goodbye to get through, one I'd been putting off because I knew how difficult it was going to be but one that I couldn't leave without. That goodbye would be a *See you later* to my best friend of nearly twenty years, who felt far more like a sister than a friend. I knew this one was going to hurt.

Tanya and I had met when we were ten years old. She was my first friend in a new school after my family moved to a rural community forty-five minutes outside Salt Lake City. She was tall and towered a full eight inches over me, so when she invited me to play at recess, quite honestly, my tiny ten-year-old self was too intimidated to say no. And I'm glad I didn't, because from that day forward, the two of us became inseparable. From lemonade stands to sleepovers, boyfriends, heartbreaks, dances, and summer jobs, we were side-by-side through it all. Wherever she went, I went; everything I did, she did. Even as we grew into adulthood, we matched each other step for step, both excelling early in our careers, buying our first homes before we were twenty, each becoming engaged by twenty-one and married shortly thereafter.

Our lives and our paths didn't diverge until my marriage started failing right as hers was beginning. I was married and had been living in Austin for a year with my ex-husband when Tanya asked me to be her maid of honor. There was no question I'd say yes; this was a day both of us had dreamed about our entire lives, so of course I was going to be there. Except due to the strained relationship between her and my then husband, he didn't get an invite—something he was seemingly fine with and we talked at length about before I left. However, while I was out of town for Tanya's wedding, he filed the divorce paperwork that we'd both filled out but agreed not to file months before. I came home from my best friend's wedding to find out we'd been divorced since Wednesday.

I stayed in Texas on my own after my divorce to try to put some time and distance between me and my ex, who moved back to Utah when we separated. We had a notorious cycle of breaking up and getting back together over and over again. Determined to break the cycle this time, I was going to need distance to stick it out. Tanya's path and mine diverged further, but our bond never wavered. She'd come to visit me in Texas a few times every year, and I'd fly back up to Utah to visit as well. We'd always pick back up right where we'd left off.

We had maintained our friendship like this for seven years until I moved back to Utah after my grandma's passing. Although we were living very different lives, our paths aligned once again when over lunch we both ended up sharing our plans to start a family in the next year—a surprise shift for each of us, transitioning from the no-kids camp we'd both been in for a number of years to the brink of parenthood. I knew this goodbye was going to be one of my hardest. I'd spent the past few months picturing our kids as best buds, growing up together just as Tanya and I had. I wasn't ready to face the fact that we were leaving that behind.

When Tanya came by, we decided to go for a walk around the block for some privacy while we talked. It was cold and snowy, but I knew walking would be the easiest way to have this conversation. Over the past few weeks, I'd developed a coping mechanism of completely avoiding eye contact anytime I talked about cancer. The head tilts, watery eyes, and devastation I saw etched on everyone's face while I delivered the news was always a crushing blow and a reminder of the devil on my doorstep—one I didn't have the strength to face. But avoiding eye contact while I delivered updates made me feel, in a way, like I didn't have to. I bundled up in my boots and a puffy coat, thankful to have a familiar setting and landmarks to look at as we walked.

We had texted back and forth while I was at MD Anderson, so she had the broad strokes of how the trip had gone. But as we walked along the snow-scattered sidewalks, I gave her the full rundown on my appointment and what treatment was likely going to look like going forward. It didn't look like surgery was going to be an option there either, but my oncologist had mentioned that I could likely get the same treatments at Huntsman as I would at MD Anderson. I didn't need to move if we didn't want to, as I could just fly down to Houston every three months for restaging. I watched out of my periphery as she nodded her head along supportively with each update, weighing in with encouragement and waiting for me to let the cat out of the bag. We both knew these updates were just a filler as I tried to gain the courage to finally say the words out loud.

I shared with her the conflict I felt, wanting to stay for friends and family but struggling to picture flying back and forth so often. I told her about the difficulty we'd had in finding housing here and the sense of dread I felt about spending my final days locked inside through another Utah winter before finally breaking the news that we'd decided to move. She'd clearly seen the writing on the wall long before arriving for our walk, but that didn't make it any easier to get out.

If there was one part of our childhood friendship that I'd never quite grown out of, it was seeking approval from the one person who knew more about me and all my faults better than any other person on this planet. Tanya knew me better than I often felt I knew myself. She'd always seen the writing on the wall before every poor choice I'd made in the past. She usually quietly voiced her opinion, then supportively stood by while I stubbornly learned from my own mistakes, but she always offered an outstretched hand to help me back after I'd fallen. But this time, I didn't have the luxury of trying again if I made the wrong decision; time was not on my side. Still on shaky ground about the decision myself, I was worried she might see this as another poor decision I'd rashly come to.

However, just like the rest of my family had before, she met me not with skepticism but with unwavering support and encouragement. She, like everyone else, could see how much I loved Austin, how much I'd been missing it, and understood the piece of myself that'd been lost since being here. I could hear the sadness in her voice, but she agreed that Austin would be the best place for Brian and me. She promised many trips down to visit, just as we'd done before. We both fell silent as we rounded the corner on the edge of the neighborhood, each holding back the emotions, knowing the minute either of us cracked, we'd turn into mascara-smeared messes.

We were both searching for a distraction, something other than cancer to talk about in an effort to hold back the emotion. Tanya finally broke the ice. "I actually have something to tell you too," she said with a mixture of excitement and apprehension in her voice.

"Oh yeah?" I excitedly replied, grateful for the shift in focus and conversation.

She smiled.

"Well, tell me!" I proclaimed, excited to finally talk about someone else for a change. For the past month, it had felt like all anyone wanted to talk about was me, and my life was awfully depressing these days. I missed hearing about other people.

No longer avoiding eye contact, I looked over and watched a smirk spread across her face as she tried to suppress it and draw out the surprise. I remembered our recent conversation over lunch. *Oh my god, that's it, she's pregnant, isn't she!* I thought to myself as I tried to read her body language in case this wasn't that kind of news. But I knew that look; she had good news, and she was trying to hide it. Tanya was notorious for never being able to control her facial expressions; she turned beet red anytime she tried. I watched as the hue of her skin slowly began to resemble a ripening tomato as she looked over. "I'm pregnant!" she said.

"Oh my god! Really?!?" I exclaimed with excitement. "I knew it! How far along are you?" I asked.

It was still really early—she was only a few weeks in and hadn't told anyone other than her husband yet—but she'd wanted to have the chance to tell me in person before I left. I shot rapid-fire questions at her, wanting to know everything.

"When's the due date? How did you tell Tyler? Was he excited? When do you find out the gender?" I got so carried away that I'd almost forgotten about the cancer entirely. That is, until I heard the due date.

Mid-August. Her little one would be joining the world in just under eight months. But eight months felt like an eternity as my mind began to drift, picturing what life might look like by then. Would I be healthy enough to travel to see Tanya and the baby? And what about her baby shower, helping plan a gender reveal, picking out baby clothes, and all the other things I'd imagined us doing together just a few months prior as we'd talked about starting our families? Imagining missing out on it all hurt. But what hurt more was the doubt that began to creep in. Would I still be alive by her due date?

I felt the tears surfacing as I tried to suppress the thoughts. I was so incredibly happy for her; I didn't want to ruin this moment. I maintained a smile and tried to stay present, focused on our shared excitement, while inside my heart was shattering. I'd never been filled with such pure joy and happiness yet so heartbroken all at the same time. I'd soon learn to become familiar with this wide and conflicting range of emotions as life continued without me.

I might not have known what the future looked like or how much I'd be able to be involved while I was undergoing treatment, but the one thing I did know was how grateful I was to be able to share this moment with her. Once we reached the house, we both slowed our pace, not quite ready to say goodbye and delaying the emotional farewell we knew was coming.

"You have to text me and tell me how your doctor's appointment goes next week," I said, attempting to shift into a casual goodbye, as if we were parting ways after grabbing dinner instead of diving into what could be a last sentimental farewell.

"I will," she said as she grabbed her keys. We lingered for a moment, staring at our feet, the door, the cars passing in the street—anything as a distraction as we avoided confronting the moment.

"Keep me updated on your appointments too," she said as I saw the tears filling her eyes. My vision blurred as tears filled mine too. "You're going to do great, and I promise, I'll come down to visit often. This isn't goodbye; it's see you later." Her voice cracked, and the tears began to stream down both our faces as she outstretched her arms and we hugged goodbye.

"Exactly. Not goodbye, just see you later," I replied, trying to pull it back together, mascara streaming down my face.

Although neither of us was the hugging type, we squeezed extra tight for this one, expressing everything we didn't have the words to say. We'd been friends for twenty years, but we'd never been the "run, hug, jump up and down excited to see each other" kind of besties. We were the "Hey, dude" kind of besties—a casual, low-maintenance friendship. The kind we knew would always remain unchanged, no matter how much time passed. We had an unspoken bond that neither of us put into words often. Instead, feelings were often wrapped in our all-encompassing use of the word *dude*. It acted as its own communication in ways, from casual greetings—"Hey, dude"—to supportive statements—"I've got you, dude."

Releasing Tanya from our hug, I let out a deep sigh. She reached for the car door and I walked back toward the house. "See you later, dude," I said as I waved a final goodbye.

"See you, dude," she replied, waving back as she climbed in and started the car. I held it together just long enough to step inside before breaking down and collapsing into a puddle of tears on the other side of the door.

With our final goodbyes to our loved ones wrapped up and all of our belongings packed into a small container at the end of the drive to be shipped separately, it was officially time to hit the road and begin our journey to Texas. I watched through the rearview mirror as the townhome and the life we'd started to build together faded off into the distance. This was it; there was no turning back now.

Our end goal was to be in Austin, where the container filled with our belongings was headed, but currently our GPS was pointed to Houston. We were still unsure what treatment would look like and how feasible it would be to live in Austin and commute in for appointments. So we'd decided to start this new chapter of our lives in Houston first, where we'd live in an Airbnb for a month or two while we waited for additional information. All we had in our car were a few suitcases, a bin of miscellaneous items, and Baxter and Dora.

Over the years, Baxter had become my travel companion. As he had traveled cross-country with me many times before, I knew what to expect with him. However, traveling three days with a cat was completely new territory and would become quite the adventure.

Bringing along a cat for a road trip meant we couldn't pack our belongings too high, because we needed to make sure they wouldn't topple over and crush her on the drive. It also meant we'd be hanging out with a litter box the whole way. Brian drove for most of the trip, and I was on cat-wrangling duty, which meant alternating between hanging out with the perfect angel cuddling on my lap and chasing after the agitated monster climbing all over everything and tucking into the tiniest of hiding spots, where she risked being squished on a hard brake. The trip was full of comical memories that we can look back on now, but at the time, it certainly wasn't our idea of a good time.

After three long days of cat wrangling, puppy potty breaks, truck stops, and roadside hotels, we finally arrived, checking into our Airbnb in Houston just a few days before my MD Anderson appointments. Our Airbnb was a one-bedroom apartment that was seven floors up and just about as far away from the elevator as it could be—the elevator that Brian memorably tripped out of after trying to take three loads in one go while already being in a grumpy mood from several days of stressful travel. After he made it back inside, we silently sat on the couch as I stared at the pile of belongings that he, in an effort to take care of me, refused to let me help with. I looked over at his freshly scuffed knee, wanting to wrap him in a hug or remind him that he should have let me help, but I knew he was still too grumpy for that, so instead I playfully joked, "You know . . . I decided to get cancer just so you'd feel bad for me and I'd never have to move heavy things again."

I watched as he tried to suppress a smirk before softly bantering back under his breath, "I knew it . . . By the way, I scuffed my knee for you. Did you see it?"

"That looks pretty painful—I'm not sure you'll survive . . . but you know, with the cancer, it looks like I won't either. Should we pick out our graves together? Date night?" I replied with a smirk, the tension in the room moments before lifting.

"Naw, not yet. I think I might pull through," he tossed back.

I made my way across the room and began rummaging through one of the bins in search of Band-Aids before tossing them his way. "All right, fine. I guess I'll have to too."

"Deal," he replied, intercepting my pass and standing up to deliver a quick forehead kiss before making his way to the bathroom to clean and bandage up.

Although I wished he'd just let me help bring the boxes in, I appreciated that he was a good sport about me teasing him. These jokes always served as a reminder that we were in this together and had much bigger foes to face than each other.

— 16 —

*I feel like I'm constantly one step behind but knowing
everything is out of my direct control. It's a hard pill to
swallow sometimes.*
—Instagram post, February 16, 2021

JUST A FEW days earlier, Brian and I had cleaned out our closet. We'd carefully separated our clothes between items that would be coming with us in our suitcases to Houston and those that would get tucked away into a box going to Austin. I noticed the growing pile of coats and jackets Brian had packed away for the latter. "You're not going to take any jackets to Houston?" I asked as he tossed the last coat into a box labeled WINTER CLOTHES and pulled a long stretch of packing tape to secure the seal.

"I've got a jacket," he replied, pointing to a windbreaker he had folded and packed into the corner of his suitcase, next to seven versions of the same T-shirt he had in varying shades and two pairs of shorts—his "essentials" for Houston.

"You can't wear shorts and T-shirts every day. It's winter; it still gets cold in Texas. You're going to freeze. You need a coat," I said, with an endearing laugh at his simplicity.

"I don't just have shorts. I've got a pair of pants," he replied.

"One pair? That's not going to cut it, and you need a coat, sir."

"I'll be fine. Texas doesn't get cold. I'm from Utah," he argued back with a confident laugh.

I tried to remind him that it occasionally dips into the thirties and forties in Texas and it does indeed "get cold," but it was a futile effort. The man was convinced Utah had already conditioned him for anything he would encounter. Utah was cold; Texas got chilly at best.

"If you say so," I said as I laughed and shook my head.

Little did he know that in about a week's time, he'd be standing outside in the snow and freezing rain in a two-hour line every day to grab us our daily two-gallon water allotment as a historic freeze hit Texas. Guess who regretted not bringing a coat?

Once we arrived in Houston and after my first walk with Baxter at our temporary rental led to a man on the corner cursing and chasing us across the parking lot, Brian suggested we find a new place to stay in a safer area. We knew the coming weeks would be stressful with scans and treatment, and we didn't want to worry about the safety of where we were living. So, with some guidance from our new friend Marvin and my stepbrother, who lived in the area, we found a new place in a quieter neighborhood with a small fenced side yard that would be safe for Bax at any hour. The following day, we packed up our stuff once again and relocated.

Inside our new townhome rental, there was a small kitchen and living room with large windows looking out onto the side yard. At first glance, the place was well kept and homey, but on looking closer, we found that the owners had a few unfinished projects underway: there were vents missing covers in the ceiling, a hole in one of the bedroom doors, a bathroom out of commission, paint samples on the walls in the closets, and a mounted TV that I was convinced was going to fall at any second, as the drywall had given way behind it. This was certainly no five-star hotel, but it was a safe place to rest our heads for the next month or two. We unloaded the pets, lugged our stuff in, and settled in once more.

The following day, Marvin and Debbie swung by to welcome us to Houston with a loaf of fresh-baked sourdough bread. They offered a few words of encouragement for the coming week and the road ahead. I shared with them the unrelenting worry and anxiety I'd been having about my upcoming scans in two days. Part of me wanted to get it over with so we'd finally have a few answers, but I also wasn't sure I had the strength to face the results.

When I'd asked about my prognosis and how aggressive my cancer was at my last appointment, my oncologist had advised me that it was too early to tell—she'd order another set of scans before I started treatment that would give us more information. In a couple days, I would be seeing the results of those scans, and even the thought of them was making me nauseous. Marvin helped ease my worries, sharing success stories of other patients he knew and all the hope he had for the new treatments that were available now compared to when he was first diagnosed. "Get ready for a battle," he advised. "The road isn't easy, but it's worth it for more time with our loved ones," he said as he looked over at Debbie with admiration. I looked at Brian with tears in my eyes.

As day turned to dusk, the sky darkened and our visit came to an end. A crisp breeze blew as Marvin, undeterred by the incoming storm, bade us farewell with a cheerful "Blue skies and clear scans ahead!" Which I echoed back as they made their way to the end of the drive. The phrase, coined by Debbie, was their cancer version of wishing good luck before scans, much in the way actors say "Break a leg" before a show.

Blue skies and clear scans ahead . . . I repeated it back to myself as if I were uttering it into reality. I clung to those words the rest of the evening, repeating them to myself again and again as a source of comfort and hope. Despite the ominous weather ahead, both figuratively and literally, I felt uplifted by Marvin and Debbie's positive outlook and optimistic spirit.

After their visit, Brian and I went to bed that evening reaffirmed in our decision to move to Texas. In Utah, we had family who could support us on the journey but here, we had a different kind of support, the support of survivors. They felt like our navigators out at sea. We were relieved we didn't have to travel this road alone, and that night, for the first night in weeks, we rested easy. Little did we know that would also be the last good night of sleep we'd get for a while.

The next morning, I was greeted by the cool air on my face and wondered if we might have forgotten to turn on the heat. I snuggled up to Brian for warmth and noticed the glow of light from his phone. "It looks like it snowed last night," he said.

I rubbed my eyes and peered over his shoulder at the screen. "What? Where?" I asked groggily.

"Here," he replied. "My service keeps going in and out, but the news here says it snowed. You should go check," he encouraged me with a smile.

"Excuse me, sir; you're the one who said it snowed. I think you should be the one to go look. It's freezing out there. I'm not getting out of these covers," I argued back.

"I know it's cold," he said. "That's why I said you should go look. I'm too warm to move."

We both knew I would be the one to succumb to my curiosity; all he had to do was wait me out. It didn't take long before the crunch of tires against snow outside caught my attention. "That sure sounds like snow," I said with a touch of childlike excitement as I rose from the bed.

Grabbing a hoodie from the floor and shuffling over to the window, I felt the chill from the glass as I lifted the blinds to peer outside. I saw a thin white blanket dusting the street below.

"Hey, look, it is snow!" I excitedly confirmed before hopping right back into bed and under the covers in search of warmth and placing my freezing toes on the back of Brian's legs as a small form of retaliation.

"I told you," he replied with a playful smirk, rolling to the side of the bed, trying to escape the icicles at the end of my feet.

Now that I was fully awake, I grabbed my phone from the bedside table to check the news. I unlocked the screen, opened a browser, typed the words "Texas snow," and hit enter. Nothing happened. I didn't have a single bar of service, and my battery was only three-quarters charged. Turns out, not only had it snowed, but the power had gone out too. No wonder it was so cold.

Brian and I lay in bed for another hour, both refusing to face the cold, until Baxter started dancing at the door, ready for breakfast. I followed him downstairs and grabbed a blanket off the couch to wrap myself in as I poured kibble in his bowl and checked the thermostat. Before bed, it'd been toggled to heat and set to sixty-eight degrees, but the power had clearly been off for a while, as it was currently forty-four inside. I snapped a picture to document the moment, still thinking this would pass quickly and the power would be back on in no time. This might be an interesting memory to look back on.

It'd be a full four days before we had sustained power again; half of those days we'd be without water, followed by a boil notice for nearly a week after that. It might look like a winter wonderland outside, but we were in for a week of hell.

After Baxter finished breakfast, I threw on a coat and took him for a short walk outside to take in the wintry landscape, survey the streets, and search for cell coverage so I could check for any updates from MD Anderson. As Bax and I made our way down the sidewalk, I alternated between watching my feet to ensure I didn't slip on the ice and checking my phone for signs of a signal. About a half a mile into our walk, I gave up hope for service and stashed my phone back into the oversized pocket of my coat, where it stayed until I felt it subtly vibrate a few blocks later.

One buzz, two buzzes, three. I reached back into my pocket and felt the vibration of each new notification coming through as I pulled my phone out and watched the display light up with a stream of notifications. There were several text messages from family and friends checking in on us and one new voice mail from an unrecognized number, which these days usually meant a call from insurance or a doctor's office. I pressed play and raised the phone to my ear to listen.

The voice mail was indeed from MD Anderson. They informed me that my appointments would be held virtually and my scans postponed to the following week due to the storm. My stomach dropped. This meant another delay in my treatment plan, which had already been postponed by over a month after the move and second opinion. I remembered reading posts in support groups about other patients' treatment plans, especially how quickly they'd started theirs, and my mind raced as I wondered what this would mean for my own plan. My case was supposed to go to the tumor board the next day so they could decide on a treatment plan for me. A tumor board that was held only every other week. Feeling overwhelmed and defeated, I began the trek back home.

Brian and I tried our best to stay occupied and keep our minds off the situation, playing hours of card games from bed and layering nearly every article of clothing we owned to stay warm. Every few hours, Brian would manage to get enough service to keep up with the news, but things weren't looking good. As the hours passed, it became increasingly clear that we wouldn't have our power restored anytime soon.

The only food we had that didn't need refrigeration was a loaf of bread, a small pack of tortillas, a box of cereal, crackers, and peanut butter. The rest of our groceries were either frozen or refrigerated, and they were getting warmer as each hour passed. We emptied the big plastic bin we had brought with us and filled it with the contents of our fridge before placing it on the patio and hoping for the best.

We made lunch with whatever we could scrounge together. For me, that ended up being a couple strawberries, some pineapple, and a cheese quesadilla. I realized halfway through sprinkling cheese on top that since the stove was electric, we had no way to cook it. I made a sad attempt at melting the cheese using a lighter without much success before eventually giving in and eating it as is. Brian, on the other hand, was much more successful with his lunch: PB&J on tortillas, which I had to admit was much tastier than my sad, cold, crumbly quesadilla. Come dinner time, we both opted for his creation.

As night fell, we were still without power and knew we were in for a long, cold night ahead. We gathered every blanket in the house to layer over top of us before turning in for the night and snuggling up for warmth. It didn't take long after the sun went down before temperatures started to plummet and we struggled to retain heat. I tried to keep my head warm with a beanie and the covers pulled over my head, but the thick layers felt suffocating. I kept uncovering my head, only to have the cold air biting at my nose after an hour in a cycle that would last the entire night. I could hear Brian doing the same from his side of the bed, neither of us catching sleep as the night drew on.

The next morning, as the sunlight began to peek through the bedroom window, I gave up on any hope of sleep and groggily got out of bed. I'd avoided showering the day before because the idea of hopping into a cold shower with no way to warm back up in a house stuck at forty-four degrees didn't exactly sound appealing. But as I ran my hands through my hair, the greasy, oily texture clung to my fingers, flattening it against my scalp. It was time for a wash. Hoping a cold shower might also wake me up, I lit a candle from the side of the bed, made my way to the bathroom, and flipped on the shower. I heard the water trickling through pipes, but nothing came out. *That's weird*, I thought, turning it off and trying again—still nothing. I toggled the divider to allow the water to flow freely into the tub, and a small trickle came out. Worried the pipes might have frozen, I called Brian. "Uhhh . . . we might have a problem."

"What do you mean?" he asked, rising from bed to look.

"I tried to take a shower, but there is only a weak stream when I switch it over to the tub," I explained while demonstrating.

"There's no pressure," he said, moving over to turn on the faucet at the sink. An even slower trickle came out. He unlocked his phone, and we both waited as a single bar of service refreshed the Reddit feed we were using for updates. Not only was most of the city still without power, but many didn't have water. Those who did didn't have pressure and were now under a boil notice.

The shower soon became the least of our worries as we realized that not only were we running out of food, but we had no water in the house and no way to boil whatever we could manage to get from the faucet. The roads were still icy and people were advised to stay inside, but we didn't have a choice; we had to try to make our way to the store. Thankfully, there was one just a few blocks away.

The drive over was terrifying, to say the least. The roads were icy and snow covered. We slid all over the place trying to make it out to the main road. As we pulled into the grocery store parking lot, we realized this wasn't going to be a quick trip. Only a limited number of people were allowed inside at a time. A long line had formed out the door, down the side of the building, and into a parking lot full of people waiting in the freezing rain. Only one of us would be allowed in, and Brian didn't want me out waiting in the cold, so he volunteered to gather water and shelf-stable groceries to get us through the week. We parked the car, and he went out with his light jacket to secure his place in line.

I felt helpless as I sat in the car. Brian had never really treated me any differently post diagnosis—he'd comforted me, sat with me while I cried, and provided encouragement—but this felt different. At this point we still knew absolutely nothing about cancer. We'd heard patients could have a lower immune system but didn't know that typically came from treatments and not the cancer itself in solid tumors. I didn't feel sick, but this was the first time I'd felt him protecting me as if I were. I felt guilty that I wasn't the one waiting in line—I was the one who'd actually packed a coat, after all. I felt equal parts loved by his protection and saddened by the thought that I needed protecting.

He made it back to the car two hours later with two gallons of water and a few bags of groceries. Most of the food had been picked over, and they were limiting water purchases to two per household. We had enough to get us through the day, but it looked like we would be back to do it all over again tomorrow. I was just grateful they'd had anything in stock and for the workers who had stayed on as part of the storm crew to ensure they could remain open for the community.

Once we made it back home, we tossed out the groceries we had placed on the porch, as it was clear they'd gone bad. We began using the large plastic bin to store any water we could get out of the faucet. We knew it was likely only a matter of time until we lost access to water completely, so we tried to collect a few pots to ensure we still had water to flush the toilets.

It took hours to fill pots with the slow trickle of the sink, but we were glad we'd gotten started when we had, because by time we had a few pots collected, water had stopped coming out of the faucet completely. We now had two gallons of fresh water, a few pots of boil-notice water, and a stash of snacks to get us through the next few days.

With the batteries on our phones running low and the lighter we had for the candles nearly out of fuel, we called it an early night, piling back on the bed with all the blankets and pets for another cold and restless night. Unable to get warm, I lay in bed, worried about the stress on my body. My mind raced all night long, which only added to my exhaustion the next day, which would go on record as being one of the most difficult days I had through my diagnosis.

The next morning, we were still without power or water, and my phone couldn't pick up a signal. We'd relied on Brian's the past few days, but this now posed a problem for the telehealth appointment scheduled later that morning. Last I'd heard, it was still on, but I needed a signal to connect. At this point, there were a couple of areas in the city where power had been restored or moved to rolling blackouts. As we checked the roll call list on Reddit, it looked like one of the neighborhoods that currently had power was in the same area as the first Airbnb we'd booked. The owners had been kind enough to refund us for the rest of the month as long as we paid through the end of the week, which meant we still had access to it for a couple more days. We decided to take the risk, venturing out on the roads in hopes of finding power and service for my appointment.

After a treacherous drive across the city, I felt encouraged as we pulled into the parking lot and I noticed a business or two with their lights on. That is, until the complex itself came into view and we heard the alarms and saw a crowd of people waiting outside. It looked like they had power, but with fire alarms blaring and half the residents evacuated outside, it was clear they were having issues with frozen or burst pipes and we wouldn't be able to go inside. I looked at Brian with tears in my eyes. "We don't have time to go back," I said, discouraged and worried I was going to miss my appointment.

"No, we don't," he said, the stress evident in his voice as he searched for a solution. "Do you have service?"

I turned on my phone, and after it booted, I swiped up to access the home screen. With eagle eyes focused in on the top right corner, I saw one glorious bar appear. "I have service!" I declared. After a series of bad luck, even the smallest of victories felt like an enormous win. I turned up the volume to ensure I'd hear any incoming call, plugged into the charger, and set my phone on the center console, where I stared at it for the next twenty minutes, awaiting my appointment.

The minutes passed like hours, and my phone never rang. I hadn't received any updates about the appointment being canceled, and I didn't want to be a nuisance by calling too early, since I knew appointments often ran behind. But once we reached twenty minutes past the scheduled time, I gave them a call. A nurse looked up my appointment; she said it was still scheduled and that my oncologist must be running behind. She instructed me to hang tight and said I would be receiving a call soon. So that's exactly what we did. We hung tight and waited in the parking lot.

We waited for twenty minutes, then thirty, forty-five, and finally an hour. Despite no call, we continued to idle the car to stay warm, burning through our precious fuel supply. With all the gas stations closed, we knew we had to conserve what we had. After an hour of waiting, I asked Brian if we should head back home. With unreliable cell service and treacherous roads, we decided to give it one more hour. The silence in the car was heavy with exhaustion and defeat.

Unfortunately, after another hour, there was still no call. Brian and I finally gave in and headed back home. I stared down at my phone in my lap as Brian drove, the occasional tear splashing down onto the screen as I tried to suppress the worries and fears of being left behind once again. Rationally, I knew this wasn't the case; we were in the middle of a historic freeze. These weren't normal circumstances. But lately, it felt like my whole world was full of things that weren't supposed to happen: my tumor that was supposed to be benign but wasn't; my liver biopsy that was supposed to be routine but wasn't; this storm that was supposed to pass but didn't. I felt like the cards were stacked against us, and I was tired.

When Brian and I arrived home, we sat down to a dinner of trail mix and granola bars in the dark. Then it was another early night off to bed as we tried to conserve what little warmth we had left. My feet dragged with defeat and exhaustion up the stairs, and as I reached the bed, a wave of emotion came over me. I was cold, tired, and just couldn't do it anymore. The move was supposed to make things easier, but our situation felt so much worse now. I'd never been this cold for this long in my entire life, I was sleep deprived, and after the missed appointment, it felt like it had all been for nothing. I wanted to go back to our family and friends in Utah. Tears streamed down my face as I realized what that ultimately might mean for my fate. But I didn't care; I couldn't do it anymore.

"What's wrong?" Brian asked, noticing me crying and wrapping his arms around me in a comforting embrace while he tried to figure out what had caused the sudden breakdown.

"I can't do it anymore. I'm cold. I'm miserable. I'm scared . . . I just want to go home," I replied as I hysterically cried.

He pulled me in tighter. "It's okay, we'll get through this," he reassured me.

"I don't want to get through this. I want to go home. I think I made a mistake. I'm afraid it's too late to start treatment. I'm scared the cancer is growing and that we've waited too long. I'm scared I'm not even going to have a chance to fight it," I voiced as I spiraled. "If I'm going to die, I don't want to die here . . . alone," I said, my voice breaking as I uttered the words and the emotion crashed over me. At twenty-nine years old, I'd never thought I'd be talking about death, and I didn't have the strength to face it. "Can we please go home?" I begged.

"We can after the storm, but I don't think that's what you want," he replied.

"I don't want to go after the storm. I want us to go now. I can't do another night in the cold," I argued.

"We can't go now. The roads are terrible, and we don't have enough gas to get out of the state even if they weren't. Every station is out of fuel," he reminded me.

"Can we go to a hotel? I can't do this; I don't want to do this anymore," I cried in defeat, at a mental breaking point. Waving the white flag, I wondered what everyone who'd labeled me "strong" would think of me as they watched me complain, cry, and so easily give in. If I couldn't handle a storm, how was I supposed to handle treatment? I didn't want to be strong; I wanted to be comfortable.

Brian knew there wouldn't be a hotel in the vicinity with power and an open room, but he humored me as we used his phone to find hotels that were within range of our gas tank's capacity. After calming the tears, I called several, looking for availability. Two had power running on backup generators but were completely booked for the rest of the week. One wasn't booking rooms because they had burst pipes, and another never answered the phone. Deep down, I'd known this was going to be a futile effort, but I wanted a way out. I hung up the phone and handed it back to Brian, defeated. There was no going home. There was no leaving. The only way out was through.

*At the end of the day when you cross that finish line . . . No
one is going to care if you raced the same line as the next
guy. Or how many times you hit the wall before you learned
your limits. For mistakes are our roadmap to success. The
important part is you made it.*
—Instagram post, May 10, 2014

*T*HE ONLY WAY *out is through.* The phrase doesn't depict
strength in a traditional fashion. It describes a singular
path with no escape routes, which feels like a fitting description of having cancer at times.

I wasn't choosing to be strong, and my actions certainly
didn't feel like strength. Every decision I made was through
a pile of tissues and a puddle of tears. I complained, I asked
"Why me," and I was terrified every step of the way. The truth
is, I wasn't acting out of strength; I was simply trying to survive. When your back is against the wall and the only way
out is forward, it doesn't matter how scared you are; you start
walking.

The path often felt reminiscent to me of an experience I'd
had canyoneering and rappelling with my coworkers several
years prior to my diagnosis. I was working for MotorsportReg,
a small startup that built software used at racetracks. It had
been my dream to be working for the company, and I'd spent
three years pursuing a job there before I ever landed one.

I've had a love of cars and for being behind the wheel for
as long as I can remember—but not in a posters-on-the-wall,

walking-encyclopedia-of-car-facts kind of way. It wasn't the gears and motors that drew me in; it was the freedom of being on four wheels, and the memories and joy it created, that formed my bond and connection with cars.

In the large family I'd grown up in, going anywhere meant dividing up between two cars, which always turned into a race, regardless of whether our destination was five or fifty miles. I'd always call dibs on riding with dad, knowing even trips to Grandma's could turn into a high-stakes road rally. With a strict no-speeding rule in place and a week's worth of bragging rights on the line, my brother and I would call out side streets and time stoplights from the back seat as we laid out the best route to ensure our victory.

When my stepsister, who was eight years older than me, turned sixteen and got a car of her own, running errands with her quickly became one of my new favorite pastimes. After carting my siblings and me around town, she'd occasionally pull off at the church parking lot down the street to let me steer and wind our way through the empty lot. We might have only been going five miles an hour, but with the wheel gliding through my little hands, it felt like I was on top of the world. I cranked and navigated the wheel, soaking up the freedom to call the shots by pointing the nose of the car in any direction my little heart desired. As the youngest of seven, I rarely got such an opportunity, so I relished every second with a beaming grin spread across my face.

I constantly begged my siblings to play round after round of N64's *Cruis'n USA* and *Mario Kart* and would try to sneak in turns on my neighbor's full video game racing setup with my childhood best friend. We'd play endlessly, until her brother finally banned us after we'd used his rally car to play house a few too many times. Driving backward on the racetrack as we pretended to drop off our imaginary kids at soccer practice had destroyed his progress and his rankings in the process.

The day I got my learner's permit, I was chomping at the bit to get behind the wheel and learn how to drive a manual. I learned and honed my skills in the car my dad had bought the year I was born—the one passed down through my siblings and held together with duct tape, staples, and glue by the time that beautiful faded-blue rusted gem made it to me on my sixteenth birthday. Frankenstein, as we affectionately called it, was my pride and joy—five-speed, six-cylinder freedom on wheels, with plenty of pep, personality, and a finicky ignition. I spent every second I could behind the wheel, offering rides to friends for gas money and taking on extra chores to fill the tank until I got a job. So, naturally, when Miller Motorsports Park (now Utah Motorsports Campus), the longest road-racing course in North America at the time, was built and opened its doors in my small town when I turned sixteen, it was the first place on my list to apply to for my first job.

I sold tickets from a six-by-eight booth in a dirt parking lot and worked my way into management with a full-time salaried position before I was eighteen. That track was my second home, and the roar of engines, cars on the track, and event announcers overhead became the soundtrack to my summers.

I loved that place but ultimately knew that ticketing and a box office manager position weren't my end goal or dream job. As much as I loved the track, I hated the confrontation that came with running a box office. Dealing with upset customers and masquerading as an extrovert always left me drained and exhausted at the end of each day. What I really thrived on was all the behind-the-scenes work that led up to event day.

With the track still building its systems and in the booming tech era of the very first iPhone, I was obsessed with finding new ways to automate and organize systems using computers and the latest tech. I meticulously combed through data and ticket sales from the system, translating the columns of messy letters and numbers into organized structures that told a story. My first year of management, I cut the budget in half by picking up on the patterns and the predictions that could be made from them.

There was something so satisfying about using tech to relieve bottlenecks and pain points for people or discover new insights no one else had found before. Through this exploration of tech and new systems, I had the opportunity to help implement one of the first online registration systems for motorsports, which is precisely where my budding itch to work in tech began. I watched how it transformed not just registration queues but the entire experience for everyone involved, giving people time back to enjoy themselves instead of wasting hours in line. I was hooked and knew I wanted to be a part of these solutions.

So when a friend asked one afternoon what my dream job would be and I answered, "To build software for racetracks," I quickly walked back my comment with "But I'm not smart enough for that." Growing up in a small town in the mid-2000s, I'd only rarely come across any software engineers. Before I worked at the track, I'd never actually talked to or interacted with any, and I was certain they all must come from Ivy League schools and tout genius IQ levels. I also couldn't help but notice that I didn't see many female software engineers.

But I knew I wanted to be involved in some way, so I figured, *Shoot for the moon and you'll land among the stars.* I might not have the skills yet to be a software engineer, but I did know MotorsportReg in and out and was one of the biggest advocates for the software. I might not be able to build it yet, but I could sell and support it. So that evening, I fired off an email to the founder of the company, asking if they had any openings.

I assumed they were a much larger company, given the level of software and support they produced, but I came to find out they had only one employee outside the founders at the time and weren't hiring at the moment. But the founder encouraged me to keep in touch, in case there were any openings in the future. So for the next three years, I did just that, following up every six months to a year to check in and see if they had any positions open, until eventually the stars aligned and I was brought on board.

Over the next few years, we added new faces and expanded to a small but efficient and established team. We all worked remotely but had team meetups twice a year where we rented a house that we'd all work from as we built bonds and connections stronger than those in most in-person jobs I'd held. We all might have lived thousands of miles apart, but in true start-up fashion, these people became like my second family. So much of who I was now had come from lessons I'd learned with and from them, including the now-so-fitting "the only way out is through."

During this particular meetup, we'd had an excursion planned to hike and rappel through the slot canyons just outside Zion National Park. I remember looking at the website beforehand, trying to decide if I wanted to do it. I was terrified of heights and wasn't sure if I physically had the stamina and capability. But my boss at the time, who was one of my greatest mentors, had taught me early on in my career that growth happens just outside your comfort zone. With that advice, I'd tackled and accomplished so many things I hadn't thought I had the ability to. So I signed up.

When we got to the canyon, the guide provided a series of warnings, ran through the safety protocols, and reminded us that where we were going there was no service, no other way out, and no way for anyone to get to us. Once we got down, we'd have to be able to get ourselves back out. My mind raced as I imagined myself stuck at the bottom of the canyon, left for the buzzards to pick over my body, but I wasn't about to be the only one to back out.

We started off with a few easy rappels to get us comfortable with the technique. They were short, maybe ten to fifteen feet, but I could feel my heart racing as I stepped over the edge each time. After making it through a few rappels unscathed, I started to build up confidence, and they became easier. As we descended farther and farther into the canyon, I was blown away by the beauty surrounding us. There were endless stretches of red swirling rock towering overhead, providing cool shade from the blistering desert heat as we hiked and waded through the slot canyons. I found myself in complete awe and reaffirmed in my decision to go through with the experience. I couldn't imagine missing out on this. The few moments of discomfort were worth every second of it for these breathtaking views.

I eased up a we made it farther into the canyon until we reached one hundred feet of rappel. As I peered over the edge and I saw the long drop below, my legs began to shake and my stomach turned. *What was I thinking?* There was no way I was going over that edge. I watched as one by one my coworkers carefully lowered themselves down and shouted words of encouragement to whoever was up next. "You're doing great." "Keep going." "Don't look down." The words echoed against the walls of the canyon, as did the cheering once whoever it was made it to the bottom.

When my turn finally came, my voice trembled as the instructor buckled me in and fed me the rope. "You're going to do great. Just step back and go slow. You've got this," he said as I leaned back and felt the tension of the rope in my hand.

"I don't think I do," I said, my legs quivering against the rock. Remembering that there were no other ways out, I forced myself to begin the descent. My stomach was in my chest and I had a full-blown panic attack as I made my way down, involuntarily letting out every curse word in the book as I tried to control the rope sliding through my hands. After what felt like an eternity, my feet finally touched the ground. I'd never been so scared in my entire life. I had a complete and total breakdown as I descended off the edge of that cliff in front of my entire team, who were also my peers and mentors that I so greatly looked up to. They all congratulated and cheered for me as the instructor unhooked me from the rope, but the adrenaline, fear, and embarrassment I felt overpowered any celebration I could muster up, and I felt the tears welling behind my eyes. I had to step away from the group to catch my breath and regain my composure.

I felt like a failure and I wanted to give up. I wanted someone to come pluck me out of the canyon and take me home, but I knew that wasn't an option. The only way out was through. So I pushed on. But that push wasn't fueled by what I considered courage at the time; it was fueled by fear and knowing that it didn't matter how scared I was, I quite literally had no other way out. I was going to have to suck it up and get through that last segment.

My coworkers tried to rally around me, but I was not a pleasant person to be around at that point. The lighthearted and self-deprecating humor I'd used to power myself through the excursion thus far shifted as I became silent and somber, stuck inside my own head. The canyon was no longer filled with breathtaking views for me; it was now a reminder of the failure I felt like I'd become, a reminder that as much as I wanted to, and as much as I tried to will it into reality, I couldn't force myself to be as cool, calm, and collected as everyone else seemed to be. My fear and anxiety were in full control, and I was frustrated that I didn't have the strength to change it.

We made it through the final obstacles, and as we wrapped up the last hike out of the canyon, I breathed a sigh of relief and felt myself coming back to life. I'd made it. I hadn't thought I would, didn't know how I had, but somehow I'd made it, and now that I knew I wasn't going to die, we could joke about it. Everyone on my team congratulated me and made a comment about my strength while I poked fun at the sheer amount of panic they'd all watched me face.

I didn't understand how or why they were calling me strong. I clearly was the weakest one on the team. No one had struggled like I did, and they weren't giving that title to anyone else. It's something I brushed off with a joke and never fully understood until I encountered the same descriptors while battling cancer. My battle has been messy, full of tears, fear, and uncertainty, and I felt so unworthy as others looked on and labeled me strong. I didn't feel strong.

But now, looking back on all that I've been through over the years, I recognize many parallels to the experiences I encountered canyoneering that day. Battling cancer is full of highs and lows. Moments you're confident you've finally gotten things under control and proud of your progress, only for plans to change as you recognize the next descent is far steeper than the one you just conquered. It's feeling like you're stepping off the ledge backward, putting your life in the hands of people you barely know while supportive friends and family cheer you on with each step you take down the cliffside.

It's being terrified every inch down, never knowing if or when the rope may give way, then finally reaching stable ground with congrats and pats on the back because "you made it" while knowing there's still miles of obstacles ahead.

It's hitting rock-bottom but looking up as you press forward to take in and appreciate the beauty surrounding you and your gratitude to be alive. Recognizing you never would have experienced the view without the drop, but simultaneously still wishing you'd never had to step off the cliff in the first place.

Over time and through these experiences, I've realized strength isn't the absence of fear but instead a product of persevering through it. The act of continuing on, enduring through the fear, and pressing on anyways is strength itself. Strength comes from the journey, even if fear is at the wheel.

— 18 —

If I can be that one in a million case once, who says I can't do it again and beat those ugly RCC stats. Aiming higher . . .
—Instagram post, March 9, 2021

O N DAY THREE of the Texas freeze, we woke up to the hum of the fan above the bed and a blinding light we hadn't seen in days. Finally, we had power back. Over the next two days, the ice on the road began to melt, making our trips to the store for our two gallons of water a little easier each day, and with the rolling blackouts and rising temperatures, we were able to keep the house above sixty degrees, which felt like a luxury. We regained access to water, which would be under a boil notice for at least a week, but once power came back, that felt like the least of our worries.

By the following week, the worst had passed, and I got ready for a full week of appointments ahead. First was my rescheduled CT scan, where we'd find out how quickly the cancer had been growing. I didn't sleep a wink that night as I lay in bed with worry and anticipation. The next morning Brian drove me over and dropped me off for the scans. I went through screening, checked in with the front desk, and was served up the thirty-two ounces of oral contrast I'd be required to drink to help them visualize the cancer on my scans before they could call me back. *This is new,* I thought, instantly regretting the thirty-two ounces of water I'd just chugged just before arriving. At my last appointment, a nurse had struggled to place an IV for me, and she'd recommended I drink lots of water and ensure I was well hydrated next time so it was easier to find a vein. Hoping to avoid being turned into a human pincushion once again, I'd taken her advice to heart and downed the entire jug of water from the giant hospital mug I'd kept after my biopsy. The thought of trying to get down another thirty-two ounces was nauseating.

The woman at the desk asked what I'd like mixed in with the contrast, providing various options ranging from soda to fruit juice. I looked at the sign listing the available flavorings, then looked down at my watch. But I wasn't checking the time. I was checking a cycle tracker to find out how many days out I was from my next menstrual cycle. Which seems like an awfully strange thing to do before ordering a beverage, but this was standard procedure for me.

Each month, beginning exactly seven days before my menstrual cycle, I had to change my lifestyle in an attempt to prevent the severe cramps I'd been getting consistently. I watched the foods I ate, the activities I took part in, and the beverages I drank. We'd eventually find out the pain was likely caused by my tumor bleeding, but this wasn't something we knew at the time, so my only management to keep it at bay was avoiding the triggers that I knew caused the pains. As I flipped to my tracker, I saw a little pink dot on today's date, a warning label that I was exactly seven days out and I needed to avoid any triggers if I didn't want to be doubled over in pain that evening.

Soda was a trigger; a few months earlier, I'd been crying on the bathroom floor waiting for the pains to pass four hours after having a few sips of Diet Coke. I also suspected sugar was a trigger after trialing how many Sour Patch Kids or other candy I could consume before the pain would appear. After a couple months of trial and error, I'd found my limit at four. So no soda, no juice; my best bet was plain old H_2O.

I took a seat in the waiting room with my thirty-two ounces of contrasty water and watched my name slowly advance through the queue of patients waiting to be called back on the TV overhead. As I nervously gazed around, I noticed a roomful of patients, all of whom appeared to be completely unfazed by their upcoming scans while they sipped their drinks, worked from laptops, watched movies, or scrolled through their phone as if they were passing time in a coffee shop. Meanwhile, I looked like I'd downed four shots of espresso as my legs involuntarily bounced and the nerves clouded my focus. In an effort to fit in and hoping for a distraction, I began scrolling too.

I hadn't been scrolling long before I heard a nurse loudly call my name from the front.

Wait, that can't be me, I thought as I checked the screen above me. I still had at least thirty minutes to go. I looked around for anyone else moving toward the front in case I'd misheard my name.

"Katie Coleman," she announced again.

Okay, I guess that is me. I had barely made a dent in my drink; was I supposed to be done already?

I picked up my cup and approached the front desk with apprehension, feeling like a child who had been caught not finishing their meal. I apologized as I reached her. "Sorry, I wasn't able to finish," I said, lifting the cup to show what remained.

"Oh, that's okay," she said as she ushered me over to an empty room a couple feet away. "You still have time to work on it. We'll be right in here," she said, guiding me into the room and closing the door behind us.

"You nervous?" she asked as she sat down and rolled over to the computer.

Clearly I don't have a poker face. "Very," I replied.

"It's okay. I'm just going to ask you a few questions, then we're going to start your IV. We'll be done in no time," she reassured me. No time turned into what felt like an eternity. Despite the endless amounts of liquid I'd drunk, the nurse struggled to catch a vein—painfully fishing on both sides until eventually giving in and calling for reinforcements, who got it in the next stick.

Now covered in bandages and wraps from the several failed attempts, I sat back down nervously sipping my drink until they called me back for the scan a short time later. I changed into scrubs, and the tech got me settled on the table with a pillow behind my legs and a warm blanket before hooking me up and stepping out of the room. My heart raced as I heard the hum of the machine and felt the burn in my chest from the contrast as it was pushed through my IV. This feeling always led my mind to convince me that my heart was about to explode at any second, but then the sensation would fade, the machine would begin winding down, and everything would be over. I sure hated the feeling of CT scans, but the short duration always felt like a pleasant surprise.

After we got home from the hospital, Brian and I binged hours of TV to pass the time until my appointment the next morning, where we'd go over the results and finally decide on a treatment plan.

The next morning, after Brian dropped me off, I funneled through the screening and up to the seventh floor to await my fate. Soon I'd be entering a room alone, where I'd be faced with processing my results and mortality while my husband listened in on the other end of the line from the back of a Kroger parking lot.

From that appointment, we'd learn my scans were still relatively stable, which was good news. It meant, at least for the moment, the cancer wasn't growing rapidly. However, we'd also learn that my treatment goals weren't meant to be curative and instead would be aimed at prolonging my life as long as possible. And just how long would that be? Unfortunately, no one knew. Due to the rarity of my case, the treatment options I was offered had never been tested in a tumor like mine before. They were making their best educated guess to select a treatment.

The last few appointments had felt like a roller coaster ride as we tried to figure out exactly what type of kidney cancer I had, which would influence both my treatment plan and prognosis. Although all kidney cancers stem from the same organ, each type is quite different from the others, and each responds differently to treatment. For example, clear cell renal cell carcinoma is the most common type of kidney cancer, making up about seventy to eighty percent of cases. It's the type most treatments are trialed and modeled after, and it can respond well to immunotherapy. The other twenty percent of kidney cancers are often lumped into a bucket called "non–clear cell" kidney cancers, all of which are very different from each other and can respond differently to treatment. In the non–clear cell bucket is everything from papillary RCC (the second most common type, accounting for about fifteen percent of cases), chromophobe RCC (accounting for about five percent) to the more rare subtypes, such as renal medullary carcinoma (RMC), translocation, collecting duct, SDH, and several others. Due to the rarity of the non–clear cell types of kidney cancer, there isn't nearly as much research on them or treatments tailored to their biology. For example, current immunotherapies can work well for clear cell kidney cancer, the type most of the trials for immunotherapy in kidney cancer were designed for. However, other types, like chromophobe or RMC, are much less likely to respond to the same immunotherapies.

At my first appointment at MD Anderson, I'd asked if I could have chromophobe renal cell carcinoma (ChRCC), since I knew it'd been listed in my first radiology report at Huntsman, but my oncologist assured me I almost certainly didn't have it. The second time we spoke, she thought I might actually have it and was looking into trials available. And now at this appointment, my pathology had been reviewed again and again by several pathologists and they'd concluded that my tumor looked exactly like an oncocytoma, a benign tumor that's not supposed to spread. Except, mine clearly had. This would mean my official diagnosis for now wouldn't be ChRCC but instead a metastatic unclassified oncocytic renal neoplasm (I dare you to say that three times fast). They didn't call it a metastatic oncocytoma at the time, since oncocytomas are supposed to be benign and metastatic cases, quite frankly, aren't supposed to exist.

Oncocytomas themselves aren't super rare, as they account for about three to seven percent of all renal neoplasms and up to eighteen percent of all small renal masses under four centimeters. But metastatic oncocytomas are extremely rare, because the metastatic piece means they have spread, which makes it cancer. There are so few occurrences of this that the number of case reports in history (most of them from the last twenty years or so) is in the single digits. The rarity of these circumstances meant there wouldn't be much to go off of to inform my treatment decisions. So my doctors decided to model my treatment plan off the type most similar to mine: chromophobe RCC. I started with a targeted therapy, which would be a pill I'd take each day to try to shrink or stop the tumors from progressing. From there, we'd just have to wait and see if I'd respond.

I tried to put on a brave face as I received the news, nodding my head in acceptance while I shattered and crumbled inside. As my oncologist left the room and as I awaited the paperwork to sign off on for treatment, I stared down at the floor, watching my tears splash against the speckled white title below. *I sure wish Brian were here.*

After I had a treatment plan, and after finding out that it would involve me taking a daily pill, which would be a targeted

treatment instead of having infusions of chemo or immunotherapy, we began to set the wheels in motion to make our way
to Austin to settle in for the long haul. I had found a ground-
floor apartment with a small dog yard for Bax in an attempt
to future-proof ourselves against stairs. And as I signed on the
dotted line, I felt a sense of both longing and relief. A longing for the life we'd once dreamed of but also relief in the fact
that even if this wasn't quite the life we'd envisioned, at least
we were regaining our footing. It might not be a house, but
it was a home. And it wasn't just any home, it was our home.
Somewhere that, after months of uncertainty, could provide a
small sense of stability in the ever-turbulent world we found
ourselves in.

Move-in day was the same weekend my first fourteen-day
prescription for treatment would arrive. I'd been warned about
the harsh side effects from treatment: the blisters that gave way
to large painful patches of raw skin on patients' hands and
feet, limiting their movement; the crippling fatigue and the
relentless diarrhea I'd heard horror stories about, causing several patients to buy adult diapers in an effort to take back control. But there were also a handful of patients who seemed to
have been spared the worst of it, who had their side effects well
managed and under control. There seemed to be no rhyme or
reason and no predicting who would get what. Unsure if I'd
be the one to draw the short stick, I decided to spend the next
two weeks trying to make the most of this time off treatment.

Before we moved, I went for daily walks at Houston Memorial Park, where I'd listen to the gravel trail crunch beneath my
feet and watch the joggers around me. I hadn't been able to jog
in over a year. I'd make it less than a tenth of a mile before my
heart rate would enter the high 180s and I'd be forced to slow
my pace. And oftentimes, anytime I'd push myself further, I'd
end up with dull stomach cramps, which in retrospect I wonder if might have been the tumor as well. While I certainly
wouldn't be keeping up with the joggers around the pond, I

was just grateful to be out walking away my worries and hoped the side effects would spare my feet for the future.

On my way home each day, I'd often turn up the music and just drive. I'd point the car in the general direction of home but follow the road wherever it took me through new neighborhoods and winding surface streets. Much like walking, driving has always been cathartic. There is something about turning up the music, letting the words and melody speak for me while I explore new roads and wherever they take me, that is unbelievably freeing. It'd been my favorite pastime since the day I turned sixteen. Except that whole "freeing" feeling sure feels a lot more free when you're on the open road and not sitting in rush-hour traffic. So I decided, before we left Houston, I would find an open road and take a long drive along the coast. Unsure if I'd ever be able to have this experience again, I wanted to go big.

I spent a couple hours on Turo, a rental car app, browsing for the fastest car I could find. I had a short list of favorites I'd love to get behind the wheel of some day. But realizing someday might never come now, the thought that I might not live long enough to afford a dream car of my own one day made me want to live as much of that experience as I could, while I could. At first it felt pretty wasteful to be looking at supercars to simply drive around the city. Rental cars were for vacations, not gallivanting around town. However, though still expensive, the rental would be less than a single doctor's appointment had ever cost me, and far more fun.

I looked at several Porsches (my favorite) and even tried to book a BMW i8, but unfortunately, on such short notice, most of my favorite cars were booked out. So I ended up landing on a Tesla Model S instead. Since I'd be on the streets, top speed didn't matter much anyway; all I really wanted was torque and the rush that comes from being pinned to your seat as you lay down the accelerator. So I booked the Tesla, and after a quick demo from its owner, I climbed in and hit the road.

While cruising along the coast, I watched the waves crash against the shore as the speakers played a familiar tune, and I found myself completely lost in the moment. By the end of the day, I was the most relaxed and at peace I'd been since my diagnosis and without a single regret.

That day would mark a turning point and begin to spark a change in me. I'd spent my whole life trying to live up to everyone else's expectations and opinions, holding back on things I might enjoy, worried what others might think. I'd almost deprived myself of this moment because normal people didn't just rent cars and drive around town. But who cared if no one else did it; I wanted to do it. And it was one of the very best days I'd had in a long time. It was time I started worrying a little less about what others thought and spent time thinking about things that actually made me happy.

— 19 —

POSSIBLE SIDE EFFECTS: BLOOD CLOTS, STROKE, HEART ATTACK, LIVER PROBLEMS AND SEVERE BLEEDING THAT MAY LEAD TO DEATH.

AFTER WHAT FELT like an eternity of waiting, worry, and anticipation, my very first treatment had arrived in a little maroon bag—with a shocking warning label. Never thought I'd be willing to pop a pill with those kinds of side effects. I placed the bag on my nightstand to come back to later that evening while Brian and I wrapped up our final packing to make our move to Austin the following morning. I was grateful to have the move distracting me from the nerves, as even looking in the general direction of that bag made my stomach turn. But that evening, Brian and I sat down, unzipped the bag, and poured the contents onto the bed.

It felt weird for such a toxic medication to come with its own version of a swag bag. Now strewn across the bed were products to combat side effects: anti-diarrhea tablets, throat lozenges, hand and foot cream, and a flip chart of side effects to watch out for. I read aloud to Brian as I made my way through them one by one, trying not to let the fear get the best of me, with little success. As I made it down the list, I couldn't stop my mind from visualizing me in every scenario. I only made it to the third symptom before my voice cracked and I felt the tears give way. Brian reached over, grabbing my hand in support and solidarity, as I continued reading through the tears.

I took a break halfway through to grab a tissue and looked over at him—unwavering in his support as always and still carrying a stoic expression. How could he be holding it together, how was he always holding it together, while I was having what felt like constant breakdowns? I hadn't seen him cry in weeks. I didn't exactly want to see him hurt, but I admittedly was starting to feel a little bitter that he seemed so unaffected. It wasn't just my life falling apart, it was our life. Did he not care?

I knew this wasn't the case; the man had been nothing but supportive, standing by my side through everything. But your mind will take you to some pretty dark corners when you face your own mortality. *How can he be so unfazed?* I wondered. *Maybe he doesn't love me as deeply as I love him. Maybe I've become too much of a burden; maybe he just wants this all to be over with.* I felt my grief begin to manifest as bitter resentment, and I knew that if kept it in, it would only continue to mount. So before moving back to the list of side effects, I blurted out, "How is this so easy for you?" The resentment seeped through my voice.

"How is what easy for me?" he replied, confused.

"All of it. I feel like I'm always crying, but you're never upset. You never cry. How is it so easy for you?" I asked, my heart breaking as I delivered the words. Nearly every relationship I'd been in before, I'd never felt like enough. I was always chasing a love the other person didn't have to give. I'd never felt that way about our relationship until now. I felt all that trauma resurfacing as I was now projecting onto him.

"I do cry, you just don't see it," he said, as I watched the tears surfacing behind his eyes. "I was crying in the bathroom just before you came in."

"You were?" I asked, now feeling guilty for not knowing. "Why were you crying?" I asked, concerned.

"Because I was thinking about you starting treatment and wondering if we should have done fertility preservation," he said as his voice began to break. "I can't picture life without you." He succumbed to the emotion and began sobbing. "If we had a kid, I wouldn't have to. We'd always have a part of you."

The weight of his words hit like a freight train. I reached over, and we collapsed into each other's embrace. "I've been worried about how difficult it would be for you if we ever did. I didn't want to leave you with a reminder of me," I admitted, pulling him tighter.

We'd both been actively avoiding this conversation, knowing how difficult it would be. But bringing it out into the open felt like it took a weight off both our shoulders. I couldn't believe that just a few minutes ago, I had been bitter with this man, worried he might not love me enough, when he'd been internalizing his grief and trying to find ways that he'd never have to live without me.

Deep down, we both knew bringing a kid into this world and into all the uncertainty in our lives wasn't the right decision for us. We'd both accepted this in our own way, but we'd never talked about it until tonight. The emotions were a manifestation of the finality of it all. Deciding to start treatment the next morning and downing these toxic medications, for us, would mean solidifying our decision and giving up on the family we had once envisioned. That night we held each other a little tighter as we drifted off to sleep.

It wasn't until years later that I had any conversation about fertility or kids with any of my physicians. None of them broached the topic until I was a few years into the clear, and neither did I. I often wondered if this was because no one expected me to make it long enough for that to be a consideration, or if I had so many physicians that they all thought someone else had done it. But navigating those considerations alone at the time was overwhelming. We didn't know exactly what was in store but were generally aware of the toxic effects treatments could have on fertility and decided together to close that chapter.

After arriving in Austin, we were finally reunited with our belongings and began gradually establishing new routines and a sense of normalcy that had been absent for months. Each morning, I'd groggily make my way to the medicine cabinet in the kitchen, where I'd pull a bottle of pills from a ziplock bag with a bright-yellow medical warning across the front. I'd carefully shake out the tiny white pill and close my eyes as I tossed it back to wash it down. At $1,700 a dose before insurance, I'd be downing over $10,000 in medication each week—a thought that made me nauseous and reminded me each morning just how important it would be for me to fight through the side effects and fatigue to ensure I never lost insurance or my job, since mine was currently covering appointments and the centers I was being seen at, something Brian's might not.

I would close the bottle and return the bag to the cabinet and then wash my hands thoroughly to ensure I never transferred toxic residue from the pills to anyone else. Then I'd make my way over to the couch for my first blood pressure reading of the day. One of the most common side effects of this medication was high blood pressure, something that'd ramped even higher for me during the first week of treatment. We'd been able to quickly get it back under control by adding in a blood pressure prescription, but I'd now need to keep a close eye on it, checking my readings three times a day.

After checking my blood pressure, I'd shower, get dressed, then poke and prod at my stomach in the mirror, trying to feel for Newman and gauge whether I was responding to treatment—something I'd obsessively carry out repeatedly throughout the day. Logically, I knew it wouldn't be growing or shrinking at a pace I could actually feel, but having a physical reminder that was always there made the thoughts nearly impossible to shake. I'd either make my stomach drop with dread if I convinced myself it'd grown, or I'd take a little victory lap in my mind if I concluded it'd shrunk. After this quick contemplation of my own mortality, it was time to start work.

Not much changed for me at work while I was on treatment other than a tendency to take most meetings off camera to conceal my bleeding gums, a rather annoying side effect that popped up for me a couple of weeks in. After just a few minutes of speaking, this side effect would emerge, causing blood to accumulate around my gumline and creating a crimson outline against my teeth that others could see. I would often break after the meeting to swish ice water for five or ten minutes until I could get the bleeding to stop.

After work, I'd lather up in sunscreen to protect my newly sensitive skin, which would burn in just a few minutes, and head out for a walk. As I strolled through the park, I'd often listen to medical podcasts or presentations on kidney cancer in an attempt to learn more. Or I'd give Mom a call when I needed a break and an escape from it all. After each walk, I'd make dinner, then Brian and I would catch up on the latest episodes of whatever show we were watching before we'd call it a night and get ready to do it all over again the next day. For months we ended up living the same day over and over, with a few doctor's appointments sprinkled in, while we waited to find out if treatment was working.

During this time I deepened my learnings about kidney cancer, the subtypes that existed, and the differing response rates to treatment each of them had. It became increasingly clear just how important it was for patients, specifically those with rare subtypes, to be involved in their care. So I took a more active role in seeking out information on my disease and connecting with a community of other rare patients online. Since my specific cancer was so rare, I wouldn't be able to find patients specifically like me. But I instead ended up finding and building deep, meaningful connections with other young women who had other rare subtypes of kidney cancer. Most of these friendships formed either through Facebook support groups or by searching Instagram hashtags. And before I knew it, these strangers spread across the country became close friends as we built bonds over our shared circumstances, unanswered questions, and the unchartered waters we were wading through together. The basis of these friendships was a shared theme of unwavering support for each other, but I had a unique relationship with each of them.

Laura was my beacon of hope. We connected after my distraught I can't sleep, am nauseous and really scared post I'd made in the stage four kidney cancer group when I was at my lowest. We'd become close friends over the years; she understood what it was like to balance and navigate treatment, side effects, and a career. Our connection would continue to grow from these commonalities over the years.

Judith showed me the ropes at MD Anderson, shared with me treatments she'd been on, ways she'd combated side effects, and how she'd always found the courage to push forward. She was a couple years ahead of me in her treatment, and she often provided encouragement about the road ahead, one she assured me wouldn't be easy but would be worth it. We bonded over our deep love for our support systems and our reasons to live. For her, that was her husband and her beautiful little girl. For me, it was Brian. The night after Brian and I had a heart-to-heart over accepting the fact that we would no longer be having kids, she helped me work through the grief. It was a pain she knew and one she and I had talked about even before Brian and I had the discussion ourselves.

Then there was McKinley Grace, or MG. She and I were the youngest patients in the stage four support group, and even though she was an entire decade younger than I, we quickly bonded over our shared circumstances. We'd both had similar symptoms that were dismissed for over a year before eventually being diagnosed with stage four kidney cancer and extremely rare subtypes. This meant we often had more questions than answers about our disease, but we navigated that uncertainty together in the form of unrelenting support for each other, a bond that ensured that neither of us would ever feel alone.

Lastly, a group of five young women with chromophobe kidney cancer (ChRCC) welcomed me in and adopted me as their own. I'd connected with this group after Kayla, a young woman who had ChRCC, introduced me to it while I was going through my biopsy and diagnostics. We'd suspected I might have chromophobe kidney cancer at the time, and so she introduced me to the group of other young patients, who had all recently been diagnosed as well. As a group, we chatted daily, learned about the disease together, and after becoming frustrated about the limited treatment options available, all began advocating and fundraising together to fund research. Even when my tumor turned out not to be ChRCC, we'd already built such close bonds that they took me in as one of their own regardless. "You're still one of us; we're adopting you," they'd reassure me when my path report came back with something so rare that there'd be no support groups or communities directly related to my type.

These friendships gave me hope and a sense of a community. While I appreciated the support of Brian, my family, and my friends, there is a unique kind of comfort and understanding that comes only from connecting with other patients, one that can't be replaced.

The closer I became with other patients, the more I got involved in the communities and platforms online. It became my sanctuary. This was the one place where I could escape and be around people who just got it—a place I wouldn't be

battered with questions about what my prognosis was, why I
still had my hair, what had caused my cancer, or whether I'd
tried whatever treatment Sarah's mom's cousin's uncle's sister's
dog had been cured by. Instead, I found a place where I could
go from crying over wondering if my husband would visit my
grave when I died to joking about all the ways I'd haunt him
if he didn't. I found a community. And through that community, I wouldn't just find friendship; I would also find a lifeline
that would change everything.

— 20 —

*You know what I'm rooting for tonight, what I believe in
the depth of my heart? That Katie is going to be sitting here,
almost 5 years from now, sharing her story and giving hope
to the next Katie or Laura.*
                    —Laura's Facebook post, March 28, 2021

I USED TO THINK cancer awareness posts were marketing fluff, campaigns done by large national brands and companies with very little of the proceeds going back to actually benefit patients. So I never imagined a cancer awareness post could change my life until March 28, 2021.

That morning, Laura messaged me after seeing a picture I'd posted of my CT scan: a black-and-white image with a large grapefruit-sized mass filling out nearly the entire right side of my abdomen. Laura had not only been diagnosed at the same age I was, but we had a similar build. We were the same height (five foot one), and our tumors had both been pretty massive when we were diagnosed. Laura was aware of how large hers was when it was found, but she'd never seen an image of her own scans before surgery. So seeing mine was like looking into a mirror and getting a glimpse for the first time of the demon that had tried to kill her.

She'd been posting on her page daily as part of kidney cancer awareness month, which is in March, and after seeing my CT scan, she'd asked if she could share my story and how similar our diagnoses were. I felt flattered. If our journeys had started the same, maybe, just maybe, I could end up in her shoes one day too.

A few days after she reached out, Laura made the post. I must have read it a hundred times. Doctors didn't seem to think I'd still be alive five years from now, a fact I'd begun to accept, but in her post Laura had written, Katie has recently started Cabo as her first line treatment, just like me. And you know what I'm rooting for tonight, what I believe in the depth of my heart? That Katie is going to be sitting here, almost 5 years from now, sharing her story and giving hope to the next Katie or Laura. I knew Laura wasn't a doctor and she had no real way to know or predict that, but reading those words gave me hope. When you've lost everything else, sometimes hope is exactly what you need to keep pushing each day. In the months to come, she'd become my first to confide in about my side effects as she offered tips and helped ensure I didn't feel alone. And through some of the worse days, we'd joke and fantasize about taking a trip to Cabo together one day if I ever reached NED (no evidence of disease).

During one of my frequent visits back to the post, I came across an unusual comment with a picture of a bright-orange GTR linked beneath it that caught my attention immediately. It was from someone named Bruce. Orange was the color for kidney cancer, and I could spot a GTR from a mile away. These high-performance sports cars weren't for your daily driver. *What an odd thing to find in the comments of a kidney cancer post*, I thought as I clicked the link attached to the photo.

It opened to a page with an orange theme, the GTR, and the words *Driven To Cure* spread across the screen. *Is this a kidney cancer site?* I wondered as I caught the FCANCR license plate on the back of the GTR. This *had* to be a kidney cancer site. Motorsports as an industry was pretty niche, so I rarely encountered anyone in my daily life who was into racing at the time (before Netflix and *Drive to Survive* finally mainstreamed

F1 in the United States). So I immediately began scrolling. I followed and clicked a few links until I stumbled across Andrew's story.

Andrew had been diagnosed with a rare kidney cancer called HLRCC at the end of his freshman year in college. His doctors told him that his cancer would not respond to any approved treatments, but they referred him to the National Cancer Institute at the NIH, where he participated in clinical trials for his disease that bought him more time.

Andrew turned his difficult circumstances into a positive by establishing Driven to Cure, a nonprofit organization that raised awareness and funds for research on rare kidney cancers like HLRCC. He combined his passions for cars and cancer awareness using his own dream car, a Nissan GTR, as a way to spread his message. Through Driven to Cure, he'd raised $1,000,000 for research in hopes of finding a cure for rare kidney cancers.

This was an organization not only for kidney cancers but for rare kidney cancers. My worlds were colliding, and before making it through the full bio, I began looking for contact information. I had to reach out. I found a Facebook link and sent off a message to someone I thought would be Andrew, telling him how I loved what he was doing to raise awareness, sharing my background working in motorsports, and asking him if they ever held any events that I might be able to help with.

It was only a few minutes later that I made it down to the bottom of the page to find out that Andrew had since passed from his cancer two years prior, in 2019. My heart sank as I read the words. How could someone doing this much good be taken from the world so young? I sent a follow-up message with condolences but further extended my offer to help in any way I could. I almost immediately received a reply.

It was from Bruce, Andrew's dad, who had taken over running Driven to Cure to continue Andrew's mission after his passing. He was the same person who had commented on Laura's post. He shared with me the events they'd attended, the awareness they had driven, and the lives they'd changed. I was beyond moved. I didn't know how I could help but knew I wanted to be involved and support the cause in any way I could. So Bruce and I scheduled a call for the following evening to chat about how we could connect our networks. And the next day, I headed out for a walk as I waited for the call to come in.

Just before sunset, my phone rang, and I picked up to hear Bruce's voice on the other end of the line. We chatted for over an hour. He shared Andrew's story with me and his reason behind founding Driven to Cure. Andrew knew treatment options wouldn't be curative for him, but he wanted to make an impact and a difference so other patients with rare kidney cancers would have better outcomes one day. He believed so heartily in this that he even donated his tissue to research after he passed. I could hear both the heartbreak and the pride in Bruce's voice as he shared.

As it started to get dark, we began to wrap up our conversation, but before letting me go, Bruce asked me what treatments I was on. I'd told him I was on a targeted treatment, something I'd been tolerating okay, but that it wasn't aimed with curative intent. He asked why I wasn't on immunotherapy as well. I shared that due to the rarity of the type of kidney cancer I had, they didn't think I'd respond to immunotherapy. He began pushing deeper. Rare? How rare? He continued to ask questions, trying to understand more about what I was dealing with. When I shared with him that I had a metastatic oncocytoma, a tumor I'd been told had been seen only a couple times, worldwide, in history, he stopped me immediately. "You need to get to the NIH."

At this point, I'd had four separate opinions: Huntsman in Utah; a community oncologist in Utah; MD Anderson in Houston; and a local oncologist in Austin. Everyone was in agreement that surgery wasn't possible and treatment options were limited. Surely the NIH wouldn't be any different, but Bruce insisted. "With a cancer as rare as yours, you're going to want to be at the NIH. They specialize in rare kidney cancers."

I hadn't entered the call thinking that when I left it I'd be pursuing new treatment decisions or another opinion on my case, but after hearing the glowing endorsement Bruce had for the NIH, I knew I had to at least give it a shot. So when we hung up the call, I sent Bruce a quick bio and summary of what I had, and he fired it straight to Dr. Marston Linehan, the chief of urologic oncology at the NIH, who'd been a renowned urologic surgeon and was an international leader in kidney cancer. His work at the NIH had led to significant advancements in the understanding and treatment of kidney cancer, and his expertise as a world-renowned physician was highly sought after. I wasn't sure what would come from it, but I felt incredibly grateful that Bruce was willing to refer me to the top of the chain.

As I returned inside, I rushed back to Brian's office, excited to share the news. I recounted my conversation with Bruce and the recommendation to seek another opinion from the NIH as I watched for Brian's reaction attentively. Over the past few weeks, I'd been back and forth on whether I wanted to stay with the current oncologist I had at MD Anderson or switch to one who was more specialized in rare kidney cancers. I didn't know if I could switch, and most people I'd asked about it advised against changing doctors within the same institution. I also worried what might happen if I brought it up, then found out I couldn't switch. I didn't want my current oncologist, who I highly respected, to be offended or upset with me. The last thing you want to do is offend the person you've entrusted your life to. We'd moved all the way down to Texas to go to MD Anderson, and I really didn't want to screw that up.

Since my cancer was so rare, it wouldn't necessarily be any oncologist's specialty, but I wanted to get as close to that as I could. If I was going to have a rare case, it'd likely help to have a team whose wheelhouse was rare kidney cancers. I knew of another oncologist at MD Anderson, Dr. Pavlos Msaouel, who saw rare types of kidney cancer more frequently. I'd watched a few videos on presentations he'd given, including the webinar I'd caught just after my biopsy that had helped me recognize the importance of a second opinion. Judith had him as an oncologist as well. She spoke very highly of how he'd managed the uncertainty and rarity of her case. His team felt like the right team for mine as well, but I wasn't sure if I could actually make the switch or, honestly, if I even had what it took to endure the discomfort that came from asking for one.

Brian had borne the brunt of that indecision over the past few weeks as I talked in circles, conflicted. He was always supportive of every decision I made, but I could tell the uncertainty and the constant change was beginning to wear on him. During one of our late-night conversations, I asked him what he would do, hoping for some clarity. But instead, he said that if it had been him, he probably would have never left Utah. He would have gone with the first opinion so as to not rock the boat and to start treatment as soon as possible. His honesty hurt and made me question my choices. Was I just prolonging the inevitable and making this all more complicated than it needed to be? His words cut like a knife.

I could tell that he was growing increasingly weary of all the changes, and based on his slow, deliberate nod, I knew this latest development only added to his exhaustion. I understood him well enough to recognize that this nod wasn't an endorsement of my newfound optimism. Rather, it conveyed the unspoken message *Here we go again*.

After observing his lack of enthusiasm, I paused. "You don't think it's a good idea," I said, trailing off.

"I just don't understand why you're seeking another opinion. You've been talking about switching oncologists, and now this. Who is the NIH? Do you even know anything about them?" he asked, the exhaustion evident in his voice.

I felt my confidence deflating. "I mean, not a lot yet, but Bruce said when it comes to rare kidney cancers, they're the best. It's where his son went," I replied, realizing that maybe, in my excitement, I'd brought it up too soon. He did have a point; I hadn't really done my homework on the NIH yet, but it felt like a promising lead.

"We looked up the top institutions for kidney cancer before we moved, and I don't remember seeing anything about them on those lists," he argued. "Do you even know if they take your insurance, where they are located, or if you have to go in person for them to review your case?"

His voice never rose, but the skepticism and weariness I sensed in his tone felt crushing. "No . . . ," I replied quietly, trying to suppress the tears and the baggage from my past relationships that I felt seeping into the conversation. One of my most cherished parts of our marriage was the fact that Brian always made me feel like an equal. He never talked down to me, never belittled me, and never made me feel like a burden or an inconvenience to his life, which was something I'd struggled with in past relationships. His questions were justified and warranted, but at the first sign of resistance, I immediately backed down, tried to make myself smaller, and exited the conversation. "You're right. I'm sorry, I shouldn't have brought it up," I said, defeated, as I shifted back toward the door.

Picking up on the dramatic shift in my mood, he added clarification. "I'm not saying no. I just feel like you're constantly looking for something else, and I wish you'd pick a path. We moved to Texas; I feel like we need to get things sorted out at MD Anderson first."

"I understand," I said, my voice barely audible as I retreated further into myself, feeling vulnerable and defeated. I turned away, my gaze fixed on the floor as I walked out of the room. I was upset at myself for not gathering more details before bringing it up. And he was right: we had moved here to go to MD Anderson. Was I just fleeing having to choose between oncologists by picking whatever solution was behind door number three?

The tears threatened to spill over. I didn't want Brian to hear me cry or for him to think he was the cause of my tears. I knew that wasn't his intention, and it would only make him feel worse. The sensation of being a burden weighed heavily on me, but I was aware that this feeling had much more to do with my past than the present situation. Seeking solace and a moment to collect my thoughts, I decided a shower would provide the perfect refuge and noise to drown out my tears.

As the water rushed over me, the tears came crashing down. The past few weeks I'd settled into treatment, and it'd been a while since I'd had this level of a breakdown, but I couldn't hold it in any longer. I couldn't shake the feeling that I needed to pursue this route. I knew it was a long shot—everyone else had turned me down before, and there was a chance it wouldn't be much different—but I knew if I didn't fully pursue this option, I'd be haunted by regret.

If it were only up to me, there would be no question: I'd pursue every last option. But it wasn't just about me anymore. I had to think about Brian too. As I thought about everything he'd already sacrificed for us—moving away from Utah, his friends, family, and hobbies, all the pain my diagnosis had put him through and all the change I'd brought into our lives—I felt selfish. He'd given up so much for me, but what had I done for him? I felt like a failure, not having anything I could give in return. Maybe this was what I was supposed to give. Even more than I wanted to live, I just wanted to see him happy. I could see how much all of this was beginning to weigh on him. I loved this man more than anything. I didn't want to risk ruining our marriage or the memory he'd carry with him through these final days. Was it time to stop and just let this disease take whatever course it might?

I pushed in and cupped my hand around the tumor in my stomach, already feeling the regret from that thought. How could I willingly just let this thing win? If this option could buy us more time, it'd be worth it. I'd have time to be the wife I wanted to be, the one he deserved. On that note, I decided this would be the last and final option I'd pursue. If they were a no, that was it—no more other options, no more opinions. I'd settle in, come what may. But also, if I was going to pursue this route, it couldn't be at the same level I'd pursued MD Anderson. I'd cast the line out and see what came back, but I would do all the due diligence on my own, bringing Brian into the fold only where he absolutely was needed, so I didn't stress him out with the back-and-forth. And I wouldn't let myself get too invested in the result. MD Anderson was the priority, and I needed to get things sorted out there first; this would have to be plan B.

The following morning, I woke up to an email in my in-box from Dr. Linehan saying he had seen a couple of cases like this in the past and would be happy to review mine. I doubled back several times; had he really just said he'd seen a couple cases like mine? I'd never heard those words before. I tried to remind myself not to get attached as I eagerly scheduled a virtual appointment for the next week, casually sharing the news with Brian.

Upon receiving this news, I decided to reach out to another kidney cancer organization I'd been in touch with several times since my diagnosis, who'd recently answered some of my questions about switching oncologists. They had created a couple of the Facebook support groups that had become important to me over the past few months and often replied to patients trying to understand and learn more about their disease. I let them know that Bruce had put me in touch with the NIH for another second opinion and that I was pursuing it but didn't plan to move my care unless they were offering a different treatment plan, so I thought it was time to make the switch at MD Anderson. I asked if they might be able to help me navigate that. They graciously offered to help, and after hearing that Bruce had put me in touch with the NIH and Dr. Linehan, they offered to fire off an email to Dr. Ball, the top urologic surgeon at the NIH.

I felt like I'd gone months fumbling around in the dark, but now I had two different organizations suddenly rallying behind me to help me get the best care. I couldn't have been more grateful for their support.

During the next few weeks, those connections began playing out. They helped me navigate a switch in oncologists to Dr. Msaouel, and I had a telehealth appointment to discuss my case with Dr. Linehan at the NIH. That call would be the first time I sat across from someone and heard the words "We've seen this before"—a statement that in itself didn't bring any new answers but brought a tremendous amount of comfort and hope.

In the call with Dr. Linehan, I found out that the NIH thought surgery could be possible. But first they'd need to check my pathology in house to ensure the tumor really looked like an oncocytoma; otherwise, it wouldn't make sense to go through with the surgery. So they'd request a sample of my biopsy that they could test in house, and we booked a follow-up appointment to discuss further once the results came back. This news brought so much hope, but it was also a hope I was wary about getting attached to.

While I remained hopeful that the NIH could provide an option for surgery, I was also mindful to proceed with caution. I could sense the optimism in Dr. Linehan's voice, but it was clear that this first call was a bit out of their standard protocol. They typically waited until they had all the results back and had a chance to fully review everything before discussing the case with the patient. But after a quick review of my scans, they had decided to hop on a preliminary call to chat. I knew they were likely reviewing my original scans, as they'd referenced seeing only two or three tumors in my liver. Dr. Linehan also shared hesitation around whether surgery would be worth it if I had more—a decision he said they'll fully evaluate with an in-depth look at my latest scans once they were able to review the pathology. In the meantime, I would wait with cautious optimism while I continued to pursue my plans and care with MD Anderson.

But the excruciating pain I'd find myself doubled over in not even forty-eight hours later would be a stark reminder of how desperate I was for a change.

— 21 —

For the first time in this journey, someone has seen my case
& they have a hypothesis on what to expect. Andrew passed
2 years ago today, before I had a chance to meet him. But
I feel like I've got an extra angel watching over me and my
journey tonight.
—Instagram post, April 21, 2021

Taking a deep breath, I curled up in a ball, clutching a scalding hot-water bottle to my lower abdomen as tears streamed down my face, trying to soothe the pain from the cramps I'd been battling on and off for years now. The pain was so intense that I struggled to speak. It felt as though someone were tearing me apart from the inside and I couldn't catch my breath. "I just want it to stop," I cried out, desperate for relief, my voice shaking from the pain. "Why hasn't it stopped?"

Despite the agony I found myself in, I wasn't a stranger to this pain. Once a month, these pains would double me over and leave me gasping for air as I'd forget to breathe. But this time it was different. The pain was stronger, more relentless than ever before, and for over an hour showed no signs of subsiding.

I'd had these pains for long enough that I'd developed a routine and process to manage them. Through experimentation, I'd learned that in addition to soda and sugar, anything with high fiber, red meat, and gluten were all triggers—as well as broccoli, avocado, cheese, dairy, and any spicy foods. The list of what I couldn't eat was constantly growing. So, as this week approached, I'd shift my diet to green beans, one slice of pineapple, plain peanuts, a small serving of unseasoned chicken breast, or a handful of olives. I'd also revise my activities to avoid the pain—no high-impact or strenuous exercise—and I'd have to lower my stress levels.

These adjustments would minimize the frequency and the duration of any events I'd end up having, but whenever they did present, I had a plan for that too. I never took any pain meds, because the pain was often gone before the medication had time to kick in. I knew they'd only last somewhere between five and thirty minutes; all I needed to do was figure out how to weather the storm. Heat always seemed to help, or at least it was a comforting distraction. I'd bought several water bladders that I had stashed in different rooms. If I ever felt the pains coming on, I'd fill one with the hottest water I could, then clutch it tightly to my lower abdomen and attempt to breathe through it for the next thirty minutes as if I were a woman in labor.

The pains would usually peak, hitting a point where they'd become so severe I'd often get nauseous and lightheaded as I began to dry-heave, and I'd wonder if I should head to an ER. But I knew they'd likely pass by the time I made it to the hospital, and surely no one would believe the severity once they were gone. I didn't want to waste everyone's time; I'd just need to ride out the pain. It'd make for a pretty miserable thirty minutes or so, but when it'd pass, it'd be like they'd never happened at all.

Except not this time. I'd tried everything, and the pain would not let up. After about an hour, we talked about going in to the ER, but I knew if we went, they'd want scans to find the source. However, my first set of scans and first appointment with my new team was just two days away. I'd seen the difference in image quality between my last scans in the ER and MD Anderson's, and I didn't want to risk a poor set of scans jeopardizing our being able to tell if I was responding to treatment or not. So Brian held me as I cried through the pain until nearly two hours later, when it finally subsided and we were able to catch some sleep.

This was something I definitely should have notified my team about, as it was bordering on an emergency. Navigating cancer is messy, and I made plenty of mistakes along the way; this was probably one of them.

I hardly ate the next few days, successfully avoiding another episode before scan day finally rolled around and we made our way out to Houston for the scans.

At the appointment, I was introduced to Leah, the physician assistant on my new team. At every appointment, I'd see either her or Dr. Msaouel. We covered my history and ran through what to expect, then she stayed and chatted a while. After discovering I worked in motorsports, she shared that her husband raced, and we reminisced over shared experiences both within and outside of racing. I remember that as she walked out of the room, I thought to myself how grateful I was for the conversation. It felt so human and real. I remember thinking she was the type of person I'd have enjoyed being friends with if I'd run into her anywhere outside a cancer center. I was surprised at how much comfort that brought to my care.

Shortly after she walked out, Dr. Msaouel walked in—he was a tall man with a medium build, dark hair, and kind eyes hidden behind transition-lens glasses. As he sat down, I asked if it would be okay if I called Brian—he was unable to join me in person due to COVID protocols. Having Brian join on a call was welcomed and encouraged. A few rings in, he picked up, and Dr. Msaouel began explaining the results of my scans.

We were six weeks out from beginning treatment and he hadn't expected to see much, but the tumor on my kidney was already responding. Several of the largest tumors in my liver had a small amount of shrinkage, and the rest of the locations were stable. This was fantastic news and meant I'd stay on the same treatment and dosage until my next set of scans. Dr. Msaouel also shared with me a change in my treatment goals, one of which was ultimately to get me to surgery. While it wasn't guaranteed—we'd need to see me get much more mileage out of treatment first—it was finally in the discussion.

I tried to temper the hope and excitement that simply hearing those words brought. Dr. Msaouel patiently answered a million questions I fired at him—everything from prognosis to pathology—and after he picked up on my interest, he even offered to show me the images of my slides, which displayed what my tumor looked like under a microscope.

Since learning about my disease, I'd become quite captivated by pathology. The slides of tumor tissue they used to evaluate and diagnose cancer contained hundreds of tiny cells that they stained with different dyes and chemicals to determine the type and often aggressiveness of a cancer. The sea of pink circles and tiny purple dots looked more like art than what I ever imagined cancer to look like, and I became fascinated with learning as much as I could about it.

Dr. Msaouel's immediate and keen sense for not only my goals but my interest in learning became a foundational pillar of trust that day. It wasn't just about treating me; he was teaching me. He was willing to share as much as I wanted to learn. Dr. Msaouel's involvement in my care would ebb and flow throughout my diagnosis over the next few years—he was always there when I needed him, advising from afar when I had interventions elsewhere—but his support for my learning was a constant. I learned something new at every appointment, which I would then branch off of and explore further on my own, deepening my understanding of kidney cancer.

Dr. Msaouel and a few others—likely without knowing it, and by simply empowering my learning through interactions like these—would eventually become foundational catalysts to the advocate I would one day become. Upon this new and budding foundation of trust, I left that first appointment with both a new sense of hope and a strong confidence in my team, a relief I instantly saw in the smile on Brian's face as well when he picked me up. After a long stream of bad news, we finally had our first win.

While the pinprick of light emerging at the end of the tunnel brought a tremendous amount of hope, it also meant we had a lot more to lose again. And over the next few weeks, I'd begin to crack under the pressure.

The further I got into treatment, the more the side effects began accumulating. I could avoid the sun to prevent the sunburns, pop an Imodium or two for the diarrhea, take blood pressure meds, and put on a hat to hide my thinning and lightening hair. But the issues I was having with bleeding began to mount and hinder my quality of life. My menstrual cycles became a nightmare, preventing me from leaving the house for longer than thirty minutes, and when it wasn't that time of the month, my bleeding gums kept us from going out. They'd started to become triggered by just about everything: a two-minute conversation, biting into a chip, a sandwich, a carrot—you name it, my gums did not like it. I couldn't contribute to conversations or enjoy a meal in public without worrying about the embarrassment I'd feel as a small outline of blood began to line my gums. The few times we went out, I spent the evening sitting in silence, waiting for the metallic taste to fade.

Overall, my side effects were very manageable compared to other patients', but they were a constant reminder that this was what life was now. Unless I made it to surgery, treatment and side effect management would become a constant in our lives until we ran out of options. And until the cancer took over. The weight of that felt crushing. Our future was hanging by a thread, and I couldn't take my mind off it.

I knew the next step was to have my biopsy evaluated by the NIH. I anxiously checked back for updates every few days. Each time I reminded myself to "play it cool" and tried my best to hide the fact that I very much was not playing it cool. It'd been over a month since my first contact with the NIH, and with each passing day, it felt like we were losing precious time or, at the very least, my sanity. Being lost in the system until it was too late was how I'd ended up in this predicament in the first place, and my biggest fear was it happening all over again. And unfortunately, those fears had started to play out.

My slides hadn't made it to the NIH yet because there had been trouble locating them. After weeks of processing and follow-up, we found out MD Anderson didn't actually have them and we'd need to put in a request to Huntsman instead. When I submitted the request, I found out that the sample Huntsman would be sending to the NIH was the last sample they had. If it got lost, there'd be no option to repeat the request, and given the complications I'd had and the fact that I was already on treatment, it was unlikely my doctors would send me for another biopsy. If I wanted a chance at surgery, these samples had to get to the NIH.

When the NIH put in the new request for my slides, Huntsman provided me with the tracking number to track their arrival. By the end of the week, when they still hadn't made it, I typed in the number to track their location. Bozeman, Montana, appeared on the screen. *Bozeman? What were my slides doing in Bozeman?* I knew the NIH was a government-funded hospital; maybe they had labs spread across the country? I emailed them to confirm.

Turned out they didn't have a lab in Bozeman. They ran all their pathology in house, in Maryland. I began to panic as I tried to uncover additional information about where my slides had been sent.

After a million phone calls, emails, and hours on hold, I finally tracked down what'd happened. Someone had accidentally swapped out the shipping label back in Utah, and the slides had been sent to a small rural hospital in Montana instead. Thankfully, I'd caught a receptionist processing the package there, and she was able to intercept it before it went down to the lab, where it likely would have sat for a while, waiting to find an owner. She printed a new label and quickly got it back on the truck before the end of the day, headed back to Huntsman. The slides would finally land in the hands of the NIH the day before my thirtieth birthday.

— 22 —

The most important things in the world have been accomplished by people who kept trying even when there seemed to be no hope at all.
—Excerpt from a journal entry, June 6, 2011

"WHAT DO YOU want to do for your birthday?" Brian asked one afternoon as we were out for a weekend drive. Since the pandemic started, weekend drives had become our thing. Brian, being ten times more introverted than I, liked that our drives counted as "outings" where he didn't have to be around people. So we'd set off on a Sunday afternoon, punch in a destination, and meander our way along the back roads as we got lost in conversation.

Since my last birthday had been at the beginning of the pandemic, this was exactly how we'd spent my twenty-ninth birthday as well. I asked for three things: a nice picture of the two of us, Chinese food from my favorite restaurant, and a long drive. We dressed up and hopped into Brian's Hyundai Veloster N. We cruised the canyon roads and snapped a few pictures in front of the snowcapped mountains before making our way back home to takeout and the best sweet-and-sour chicken in the country—or at least the best one my biased palate had been enjoying since I was five. Those memories felt like such simpler times, which in itself is such an odd thing to say about anything from 2020.

I'd always imagined I'd do something big for my thirtieth birthday—a big trip or party to distract from the disappointment that came with aging. Thirty had always felt old, and I felt a mounting pressure as each year passed and I hadn't met whichever of life's milestone I should be at. I'd thought I'd feel like an adult by now, but honestly, deep down, I still felt like a child. Thirty now felt like mourning simultaneously the passing of my twenties and my youth and the "adulting" era I'd never have. No kids, no baseball games, no piles of endless laundry. No watching our little one take their first steps or the longing looks we'd cast as they drove off with our hearts to college. This was a birthday I didn't feel like celebrating but one I also acknowledged could be my last.

At every doctor's appointment I sat in, no one was willing to give a prognosis—understandably so, for a variety of reasons, but mainly because of the rarity of my cancer. No one had a clue what to expect. However, I did have a local oncologist who eventually gave me an approximation due to my relentless asking. Their best guess was that I wasn't going anywhere in the next six months to a year but that they couldn't promise much after that. This matched up with the somewhat old and out-of-date Google search results I'd read that gave spread to the liver an eighteen-month prognosis. "Eighteen months" lingered in my mind like a doomsday clock—which is probably the very reason physicians don't like to give such predictions in the first place. At times, it was anxiety producing; at other times, it felt like a challenge I was determined to beat.

Every time I asked "What's my prognosis?" what I really wanted to know was:

- Should we buy a house?
- Should we move closer to family? (If I had three to six months, yes; if I had years, no)
- Are the side effects worth it? (If it buys me three months, no; if it buys me a year or two, yes)

- Can we have kids?
- Should I stop saving for retirement?
- Will I have time to travel?
- Should I keep working?
- Do we try to preserve fertility?
- Do we put off the adoption of a new family pet?

If I had three months to live, my life would look very different than if I had six months, and six months would look very different from two years. Two years would look different from five, and on we go. Being diagnosed in the decade of decision and not having any answers to make those decisions with felt debilitating.

There were so many unknowns, and making any decision felt impossible without some type of time frame or prognosis. And it put an added pressure on birthdays, holidays, and anniversaries, as we never knew if it would be the last.

Brian, who hated taking pictures, groaned as he poked fun at my only birthday request. "Photos? Plural?" he joked, trying to keep me grounded and my mind from wandering.

"Yes, plural. It's my only birthday wish, so I mean, you're kind of not allowed to say no," I tossed back with a smirk.

"Oh, is that so?" he replied.

"Yep. Rules are rules. We're going to take photos. All the photos. So many photos. You're going to love it," I playfully insisted.

"I sure must love you," he rebutted.

"You must." I hugged his right arm, which was draped over the console between us, and leaned over to place a kiss on his cheek.

Both a playful eye roll and smile spread across his face. "Pictures it is."

Little did I know, he had far more than pictures planned for the big day.

I woke up the morning of my thirtieth birthday and opened
Facebook to see the notifications maxed out. Friends, family,
and acquaintances had wished me a happy birthday, alongside
a stream of donations for my birthday fundraiser for chromophobe kidney cancer research, which was now up to $5,000.
My eyes instantly began to fill with tears.

Frustrated by the lack of treatment options for chromophobe patients, Catherine, one of the women from our Chromophobe 6 group, had begun working with an organization
to establish a grant specifically for research on chromophobe
RCC. She kicked everything off, then as a collective, the six of
us began fundraising toward the grant together, which needed
only $50,000 to fund an entire year's worth of research. Since
I didn't have chromophobe RCC myself, I knew any research
that came out of the grant would be unlikely to impact me. But
during a time when I was left feeling isolated and alone, with
a cancer no one seemed to know anything about, these ladies
provided me with a sense of community and a bond of friendship that kept me pushing. I knew what I had was too rare for
it to be the focus of research itself, so I'd joined forces with
these women instead.

I'd watched other people run birthday fundraisers giving to different charities, and they usually raised anywhere
between $50 and $250. Since I'd never done a fundraiser before
and the idea of asking people for money was far beyond my
comfort zone, I expected mine would be the same. I couldn't
believe not only how generously people were giving but also
the incredibly kind words people were sharing with it.

Brian walked in as I was scrolling through the notifications, and I looked up at him with disbelief. "What's it at?" he
asked, catching a glimpse of the page over my shoulder as he
walked by.

"Five thousand," I said, the astonishment and emotion
clear in my voice.

"That's amazing!" he replied.

"I know it is," I said as a tear rolled down my cheek.

Brian tilted his head, trying to get a better look at my eyes, and asked with a gentle laugh, "But you're crying?"

I replied with a chuckle of my own, acknowledging the irony of the situation. "People are just so nice. I didn't think they'd care, but they care!"

"It's almost like people don't hate you!" he joked, smirking before going back to brushing his teeth. "Let's get ready; I have a surprise."

Brian told me to dress for a hike before we hopped in the car on our way to our surprise destination: Hamilton Pool, arguably one of the most beautiful hikes in the area, since it led to a stunning waterfall at the end. I'd talked about this hike since before we'd moved here, so I couldn't believe he'd not only remembered but had booked us tickets that required reservations several weeks out. I could not possibly have imagined a better morning, and the day only got better from there.

After wrapping up the hike, we grabbed lunch before getting ready to head down to our reservation at a luxury resort Brian had booked us for the night. The giant glamping-style safari tents that sat alongside the San Marcos River were complete with a spacious wraparound porch, kitchen, full bathroom, soaking tub, and vintage-chic decor—a far cry from the camping I was used to. I hugged Brian as he walked through the door with our suitcases. "This place is incredible," I said, looking around in awe.

The rest of the afternoon and evening were filled with some of my favorite things—being outdoors by the water and cooking dinner around a campfire. We strolled through the acres of pecan groves, skipped rocks along the river, and swayed back and forth on a webbed rope swing beneath a large Texas oak tree. I couldn't believe this was real life; I wished I could live in the moment forever and just forget about the cancer. I closed my eyes and felt the gentle breeze on my face as Brian pushed me on the swing, thinking this just might be the happiest day of my life. I felt overwhelmed with gratitude for even being in a place where I could experience the moment.

However, the more magical these moments felt, the more the intrusive thoughts threatened to steal away any solitude that might creep in—thoughts reminding me that these moments were the good days in the making. The ones that would turn into the memories we'd look back on and cling to when things got tough and the ones Brian would carry with him when I passed to remind him of better days.

I opened my eyes and looked up at Brian, who was guiding the swing with an endearing smile across his face, the bright-blue sky surrounded him. It didn't matter what was to come; this moment was everything, and I was going to cherish every second of it.

That day would end up being one of the best days of my life and a memory that I still hold dear. It'd also kick off a milestone in my advocacy—raising over $6,000 for chromophobe kidney cancer through my birthday fundraiser, a number that left me truly humbled. It became a day with many reminders of my own mortality but also one that showed me the beauty in the time we do have, the people who support us, and the ones we get to make and share these moments with.

I carried this renewed perspective with me into the following weeks while I waited to hear back from the NIH after they'd reviewed my pathology. The nerves mounted as I refreshed my email endlessly until I finally saw the message roll in: Your results are back, and we have an appointment scheduled to review them with you Wednesday. I felt my heart racing in my chest as if I were sprinting around the room, and metaphorically, I was. My mind was racing with excitement. The appointment was nearly a week away. I'd have to find some way to contain the nervous energy until then.

I filled the week with walks around the park, work, board games with Brian, and endless hours of Netflix until Wednesday finally rolled around. That morning as I got ready, I remembered the advice "Don't look like you're dying." Like the stereotypical programmer's closet, my wardrobe was filled with T-shirts and hoodies. I had one "nice outfit" I'd been wearing to appointments, but I had a follow-up for my bleeding gums scheduled the next day at MD Anderson, so I browsed and pushed around the hangers in search of another option.

I had never been one to enjoy shopping, and I can't match an outfit to save my life. Whenever I ventured out of my T-shirts and hoodies, I'd either end up in a dress, because it was easy and I wouldn't have to coordinate any colors, or I'd send pictures to Tanya from the fitting room so she could tell me what matched and what didn't. I pushed back another hanger, revealing a salmon-pink shirt tucked in the corner, and remembered the outfit I'd sent her a few weeks prior as I was trying to decide what to wear for a feature about me in *Health Monitor*—one of those magazines you see in doctor's offices while you're passing time in the lobby. They'd wanted to do a photo shoot and I hadn't had anything to wear, so I'd ventured to the boutique down the street, where they helped style an outfit for me. They picked a salmon-pink crop top that I felt was missing half the shirt and paired it with high-waisted jeans, a brown belt, and a pair of gold earrings. I'd thought it was cute when I tried it on, and it won Tanya's approval too, but I was too far out of my comfort zone to wear it for the magazine article. So I'd stashed it in the back of the closet, where it'd been living since. However, the best part of this being a telehealth appointment was that they'd only see the top of the shirt; I wouldn't have to worry if I got the rest right. I grabbed the shirt, jeans, belt, and earrings, curled my hair, and plopped down in front of the computer, waiting for the call.

Minutes passed like hours as I stared at the message on the screen—*Someone in the meeting should let you in soon*—nervously clicking and swirling my pen as the nerves mounted. *Define soon*, I thought. My only means of defining what exactly *soon* meant in any medical context had been watching other patients shuffle in and out of the lobby and estimating their wait times and mounting frustrations— something you can't do in a virtual waiting room. So I'd just have to sit here, twirl my pen, and wait for my future to unfold.

Suddenly, I saw the loading icon pop onto the screen, and Dr. Webster, the fellow on my case, appeared. We recapped my history and chatted about possible options they were thinking about before Dr. Ball, the surgeon who would be doing the kidney removal if surgery was possible, joined the call.

He told me they'd reviewed my pathology in house and the tumor looked like an oncocytoma, which meant that after reviewing my scans and discussing the options as a team, they thought surgery could be possible. Dr. Ball tossed in a few disclaimers and acknowledged that what I had was so rare that suggestions anyone made on my case were educated guesses, but because oncocytomas, even in the few metastatic cases they'd seen, typically aren't aggressive, he felt that "if we can cut this thing out, we may be in really good shape."

I could hear the optimism in his voice, something that was rare to hear in anyone discussing my case, and felt like my heart was going to leap out of my chest in excitement. He delivered the news with such a straight and professional face that I tried my best to suppress and contain my excitement, certain there was a *but* or a catch coming.

Dr. Ball made it clear that the surgery would be high risk. They'd likely need to remove my entire kidney along with the tumor; since my tumor was so large, it had practically engulfed the whole thing. They still had to confirm with the liver surgeon that operating on my liver would be possible as well. But they saw a path forward, and one they thought might have the potential to offer me a cure. *Cure? Did he just say cure?!* There had to be a catch. No one was offering a cure. I continued to push with questions.

My case was so rare that all the discussions were laced with questions and stipulations that made it clear this was anyone's best guess. They didn't know if surgery would help, but they were hopeful it could. In the middle of the call, Dr. Ball stepped away to consult with Dr. Hernandez, the other surgeon who'd be operating on my liver and would need to give the go-ahead on my surgery, while Dr. Linehan joined the call to discuss my case further.

I could feel the emotion in everyone's voice, a mix of apprehension and hope. The optimism never showed on their faces—Dr. Webster was the only one I could get to crack a smile—but I could hear it in their voices. They wanted to do this surgery. They were nearly certain they could do it and were reasonably confident this was the best route forward, but they had no data or evidence to back that up, which was where the apprehension crept in. *What if their instincts are wrong? What if the surgery makes things worse? What if there are complications?* It was clear we were in a high-risk, high-reward situation in completely unchartered waters, and we all collectively would need to decide if surgery was worth it.

After a quick review with Dr. Hernandez, Dr. Ball rejoined the call. An ever-so-slight smile spread across his face. "I just spoke with Dr. Hernandez, and he agrees. He thinks the surgery is doable," he advised. I felt the optimism growing, but I remained skeptical and cautious about getting my hopes up. Surely they had to be missing something. I remembered my first conversation with Dr. Linehan where he'd mentioned two lesions in my liver when I knew I had more. I drilled in further with questions. Had Dr. Hernandez had a chance to review my scans? Had he seen all the tumors? Was he sure he could get them all?

Dr. Ball confirmed they'd reviewed the scans together, and the radiologist had marked the largest five lesions. Taking all that into account, they were still optimistic that they could make this work. They had to cross some *t*'s and dot some *i*'s, but we had a path forward if I wanted to pursue it. I'd get more information in the following days as they talked among themselves and worked out the final details, but tentatively, it looked like they could do surgery around August. Which, from May, felt like a million years away, but for the first time, we had options, tangible options.

I tried to contain my excitement on the call to stay focused on my questions, but the second we hung up, I spun toward Brian with a mixture of shock and joy dancing across my face. "Did you hear that? I might not die!" I exclaimed, the playful tone barely concealing my cautious relief. "Guess this means you just might have to get used to me," I teased as the dark humor bubbled up laughter between us.

I'd found that others often didn't understand the humor I found in these moments. Everyone took cancer so seriously, and I mean, rightfully so. It's a devastating disease. But injecting a bit of lightheartedness into the stress and unknown of it all became my favorite coping mechanism, one Brian and I often bonded over. We rarely found ourselves in any situation these days where we couldn't pull a good joke out of it. Sometimes I'd even take it too far and hurt my own feelings—which in turn would give me a good chuckle. We could either laugh at the situations we found ourselves in or cry; we usually found ourselves somewhere between the two. When you've lost all else, laughter really can be the best medicine.

"But I'm not getting my hopes up," I clarified, a sheepish grin tugging at the corner of my mouth.

"Yeah, okay," he replied, eyebrows raised in mocking disbelief. "You sure about that?" He chuckled affectionately.

"I'm not, I promise!" I insisted.

He cocked his head to one side with a playful smirk.

"Okay, maybe a little bit. But just a little bit. It's not guaranteed. I know that it could get taken away. I won't get my hopes up until we know for sure. I promise."

"I know," he said, "I'm just giving you a hard time." He stood up to head back to his office so we both could get back to work, but not before we exchanged a tight, hopeful embrace.

As he left the room, I immediately sent a quick message to Bruce with the update (The NIH wants to do surgery!!!), the biggest thank-you, and a promise to call him that evening with details. Then I kicked on my cancer jams playlist, heading straight for "High Hopes" by Panic! at the Disco. As the beat picked up, so did my little celebratory jig and fist pumping from my chair now that I was alone. I sang under my breath, becoming more animated with each verse. Before the song's end, I'd find myself belting it out with tears of joy and relief streaming down my face.

As the song ended, I heard Brian shouting from the other room and erupting with laughter. "Not getting your hopes up, huh?"

"Of course not," I shouted back. "Very unfazed over here. You hear nothing . . . I'm working," I replied, chuckling as I turned down the volume.

If I were stranded on the metaphorical cancer island and could only take three things with me, they'd have to be Brian, my favorite sidekick; dark humor to keep us entertained; and music to dance through the storm to. I'd always had a deep love for music and had gone through my phase with just about every genre under the sun. As a nineties baby, my favorite activity as a kid had been annoying my brother on long car rides while I sang Britney Spears at the top of my lungs. And if it wasn't Britney, it'd be something about a barbecue stain on a white T-shirt while my aunt hauled my cousins and me around in her minivan after school; Jimmy Buffet anytime we were with Dad; Shania Twain between pickups and drop-offs with Mom. Through middle school, high school, and college, I'd cycle through hip-hop, R&B, techno, and rap before settling into my emo phase of heavy metal, screamo, and punk rock. It paired well with my dyed jet-black hair, purple highlights, gauged ears, and a lip piercing I'd done myself with a sewing needle and tried to conceal from my parents through my rebellious phase.

There is something all-encompassing about music. I loved how, no matter the genre, music has a way of connecting people through the shared human emotions that resonate with us all. A guitar solo could invoke the same feelings in me as I'd witnessed in my mom as she sang along to Shania Twain. At a very young age, music became my outlet to process and express emotion. So what better way to celebrate this renewed sense of hope than belting it out while I danced in my chair the rest of the afternoon, blissfully unaware of the whirlwind of stress-inducing decisions awaiting me in the days ahead.

— 23 —

Hang in there. You have an army of support behind you.
Thinking about you.
—Text message from Bruce, June 15, 2021

A s surgery shifted from a distant hope to a tangible possibility, I now grappled with the challenge of reevaluat-
ing my care at MD Anderson and determining their role in
this new scenario. Asking for a second opinion was awkward,
uncomfortable, and always felt like a breach of trust even if
it wasn't. If we went through with this surgery, it would be
done in Bethesda, Maryland, at the NIH. They'd indicated
they would follow me closely after surgery for any recur-
rences, but what did this mean for my care at MD Anderson?
I didn't know what the future held, but one thing was clear: I
didn't want to lose the oncologist I had fought so hard to have
on my team. If I ever had a recurrence or needed to be back
on treatment, I knew Dr. Msaouel would be my first call. Having the right people on your team isn't just about having them
there when things are actively going wrong; it's just as important, if not more so, to have them there proactively too, standing by to order tests, formulate a plan, and jump into action
when necessary.

I also trusted Dr. Msaouel's opinion and wanted to ensure
he too thought this was the best path forward. So I fired off

an email to him, letting him know about the new options that had opened up at the NIH and requesting his expertise and opinion. I wanted this tumor out of my body more than just about anything in the world, but I was still somewhat uneasy about the NIH. After hearing so many *Nos* everywhere else, I wanted to ensure they were evaluating the full picture and surgery made sense.

That afternoon, Dr. Msaouel called to discuss my options going forward. He seemed surprised to hear I'd gone to the NIH, and I couldn't blame him. I mean, I'd just switched to his care a few weeks prior. He reiterated that his aim was ultimately to get me to surgery as well and that he'd like to see me continue on treatment with the goal of having my surgery done at MD Anderson. But I knew the surgeons at MD Anderson still weren't comfortable operating; they needed to see additional shrinkage and see a few of the lesions disappear before they'd be willing to operate.

I felt comfortable with my care at MD Anderson—I trusted my oncologist, and it was a world-renowned center. I'd heard great things from Bruce about the NIH, but I didn't have much to go off of besides that. At the time, the NIH didn't have the marketing resources or a particular informative website like many other cancer centers had, so it was difficult to find additional information. I felt a pit in my stomach. *Do I roll the dice and see what happens, hoping to make it to surgery, or do I go with the surer bet and risk losing my oncologist by going against his recommendations?* I now know that never would have happened, but at the time, horror stories I'd heard from other patients about losing their providers in similar scenarios haunted me. That was something I didn't want to risk. Sensing the hesitation in my voice, Dr. Msaouel told me to take my time to think about it and he would call me back later that evening to touch base.

I felt sick to my stomach the rest of the afternoon, playing out every option and scenario in my mind. I knew what

I wanted: I wanted surgery. I just didn't want to lose my care team in the process. The other piece that came into play was knowing that there was a lab at the NIH where I knew they'd be studying my tumor. This was important to me, in case it could lead to research or insights that might help someone else one day. I would later learn that MD Anderson has programs set up for this as well, but that wasn't information I had at the time.

So when Dr. Msaouel called back later that evening, I finally got up the courage to stop beating around the bush and be frank. I told him I wanted to get my surgery at the NIH, that I didn't want to roll the dice and risk losing the option at MD Anderson, and the only reason I had hesitation was that I didn't want to lose him as my oncologist in the process.

I felt the conversation and energy shift. Understanding my goals and motives now, Dr. Msaouel reassured me that I wouldn't lose his team. He was more than willing to manage my case regardless of where I ended up. His goal was to get me to surgery too, and if the NIH was ready to proceed and MD Anderson wasn't, he encouraged me to seize the opportunity. He promised to help coordinate and manage my care, provide support up to the surgery, then continue with any follow-up and management I'd need afterward.

After that conversation, I breathed a sigh of relief, and my focus shifted entirely to preparing for the surgery—which was approaching faster than any of us anticipated. Just a few days later, I found out that the NIH bumped up the surgery to the end of June. In just three weeks, I had to be ready for surgery. This meant that I'd needed to stop treatment immediately and begin preparing for a whirlwind of appointments and other preparations. Brian and I would also need to secure housing for recovery, figure out what we would do with the pets, and give notice at work for the several weeks we'd both be stepping away. It felt like we'd shifted from a standstill to full speed ahead, and there wasn't a moment to spare.

The next few weeks were incredibly stressful and filled with taking meetings from waiting rooms, attending tele-health appointments on lunch breaks, and working after hours to catch up on anything missed during the frenzy of planning and preparing. I felt guilty for the time I'd need for surgery, knowing I'd be out for nearly two months. I only had five weeks left of FMLA (Federal and Medical Leave Act) leave, and I knew I couldn't risk losing my insurance, so I tried to do everything I could to avoid taking time off. But as I was stubbornly trying to push through, my coworkers were sending care packages and offering to chip in vacation days to cover any PTO I'd need. After their relentless insistence, I finally started to take them up on their offers. As difficult as it was to accept the help, I knew I needed it. Brian and I had so much uncertainty ahead of us, and I became increasingly conflicted every time I sat down at the computer.

This surgery was high risk, and after reading in one of my reports that my team was preparing resources to fall back on in case of a catastrophic bleed, I couldn't stop the intrusive thoughts. If things went south during surgery, was working really how I would have wanted to spend my final days? Adding a few extra lines of code to a project that someone else would come along and replace someday? Or worrying about insurance instead of spending time with Brian, strolling in the park, and taking in the warmth of the sun on my skin? Setting aside an afternoon or two with Brian or taking a nap in the hammock sure sounded like a nice way to appreciate and make the most of the time we had. I was grateful my coworkers had pushed me to take the time and step away.

In the midst of preparation, I received a call informing us that I needed to arrive to Maryland early for additional testing for my bleeding disorder. That testing would determine whether or not it'd be safe to go through with the surgery. Although we'd received the green light from the surgeons, I still needed to be cleared by hematology.

The week prior, I'd had my first telehealth appointment with Dr. Kalsi, the primary hematologist on my case. In order to properly assess my bleeding risk, we had to do a full run-through of my history, from childhood to the events leading up to my diagnosis. The empathy she showed was palpable as she intently listened, and once we reached my diagnosis, her eyes filled with tears as she apologized for the missteps and failures in the system that had led me here. It was the first time a doctor had acknowledged the struggle and delay I'd faced leading up to my diagnosis. I didn't realize just how impactful that acknowledgment would feel until that moment as our tears met. I didn't need to explain my worries or my persistent follow-up; she simply understood, and I could sense her determination to do anything in her power to ensure that nothing slipped through the cracks again.

As more preop results rolled in, it became clear that I'd need additional testing for my team to pinpoint my bleeding disorder and keep me safe through surgery. So I'd have to leave Brian behind to finish up preparations at home for a few days while I headed out to the NIH for more labs.

Outside the night I was admitted after my biopsy, Brian and I hadn't spent more than twelve hours apart since we'd moved in together a year and a half ago. He'd become my security blanket, and the thought of traveling across the country without him to undergo testing that would decide if we could go through with this surgery felt impossible. But we didn't exactly have a choice. We needed this testing before the operation or the chances of me having a catastrophic bleed from it would be too high, preventing us from proceeding.

When I touched down just outside DC, Bruce was waiting at the terminal to pick me up, and after hearing I hadn't eaten all day, he insisted I join him and his wife for dinner at their home. I was smack-dab in the middle of the week where I had to eat a modified diet or suffer through my monthly severe abdominal pains, but I also didn't want to turn down such a generous offer. "Dinner sounds great."

As we pulled into the driveway and made our way to the front door, I stared up at the elegant redbrick colonial home. I'd been to the East Coast only a handful of times, but I'd always been captivated by the fascinating architecture, which was full of character and different from anything back home. It was as if each brick and creaking board were full of stories to tell. As Bruce cracked open the door, I saw a black snout nuzzle its way through before it swung open, revealing Bruno, the family's tail-wagging black Lab mix eagerly awaiting his arrival.

Bruce stepped inside, then grabbed a treat and passed it over to me. "Give this to him, and you'll be his best friend," he advised, giving Bruno a pat on the head.

I stretched my hand toward Bruno, who cautiously looked up at me before accepting my peace offering and proposal to become besties. I gave him a little scratch behind the ears as he chomped down. "We're buds. He's going to have to come home with me now," I joked as his wet nose scoured my hands for more.

I loved Labs and had been begging Brian for one for the past two years. I'd finally convinced him back when we were building our house in Utah. As we'd toured each home, he'd even begun surveying every lot to ensure that any future pup would have plenty of room to run—a seismic shift for the man who "wasn't a dog person" when we first met. Given the predicament we found ourselves in, any new additions to our family were indefinitely on hold, so I'd have to live vicariously through others with pets. With the newfound friendship I'd won through two Milk-Bones, Bruno would be my pal the rest of the night.

Sarah, Bruce's wife, introduced herself as she welcomed me into the kitchen to make a plate of food. "Nothing fancy," she said, gesturing toward a pot full of rice and a pan of chicken on the stove. "A simple dinner tonight, but please take as much as you'd like," she encouraged.

A family-style helping of green beans, fluffy white rice, and freshly shredded and unseasoned chicken sat on the stove—the very foods that were the staples in my diet during these weeks and some of the only ones I could tolerate without pain. "This is perfect. Thank you!" I expressed as I piled a large stack of green beans onto my plate. I was relieved to have options I could eat so I wouldn't have to push my food around the entire evening, hoping no one would notice. I followed Sarah and Bruce back into the living room, where the three of us sat around the TV to eat and catch up. This was the first time we'd met in person and the first time I'd even had a conversation with Sarah, but they felt like family as they shared about Andrew and the NIH and offered well wishes for my upcoming appointments. Though I was a thousand miles away from anyone or anything I knew, their warmth made me feel at home.

As it grew dark and the sun began to dip, Bruce offered to take me out to see the GTR, which was stored in the hauler outside their house, before dropping me back off at my hotel. He lifted the door, unveiling the bright-orange car I'd seen in the photo from the comment on that very first post. "Let's take a picture," he said, encouraging me to stand beside the car as he pulled out his phone. "Ah, but wait, we're missing something," he said, stepping behind the trailer and popping the shell on the truck. "What size do you wear?" he asked as he began rummaging through boxes.

"Probably a medium or a large," I said by default, forgetting the weight I'd lost in the last year. He looked back at me, confused.

"Definitely not large. Here's a medium; see how that fits," he said as he tossed me a shirt with the organization's well-known orange FCANCR license plate on the back. I held it up in front of me as we both gauged its size. "That still looks too big. Let's get you a small," he suggested, pulling two more shirts out of the box. "What about a jacket? You need a jacket too," he insisted.

"Wow, thank you. These are great," I said softly, turning the shirt side to side to get a look at the designs. "How much do I owe you?" I asked.

"Nothing." He stepped up onto the bumper of the truck and shifted boxes around in search of the jackets.

"No, I can't take these. That's too much. I want to pay for them," I insisted.

"Nope. You're good. They're yours," he said matter-of-factly in a tone reminiscent of my dad's anytime I'd insisted on paying for dinner. "Now, what size does Brian wear?" he continued without missing a beat, determined not to entertain my idea of paying for anything.

"He wears a large. But really, I'd love to pay for them," I declared, giving it one last shot.

"Nope. Your job is just to get through surgery," Bruce insisted as he pulled out another shirt and jacket for Brian and stacked them on top of the growing pile of Driven to Cure merchandise cradled in my arms.

I graciously thanked him over and over for his generosity as we loaded into the car and made our way to the hotel. With my family on the other side of the country and Brian still in Texas, I couldn't have been more grateful for their hospitality and support. In a world of unknowns in the coming days, Bruce's fatherlike presence and support served as a stabilizing force and comforting anchor.

The next morning, it was time to head over to my appointments at the NIH. I threw on my new Driven to Cure jacket and went to the hospital. If I'd thought the screening at MD Anderson was intense, this was next level, which made sense, given that it was a government facility. But I'd never imagined I'd be walking through metal detectors on my way to having labs drawn.

Inside, the large open atrium was bustling, but in a much different way than I'd seen in other hospitals and cancer centers. Instead of being filled with patients, it was mostly filled with doctors, nurses, and staff intermingling with the few patients who were there grabbing breakfast or killing time before their appointments. I'd never seen these sorts of interactions in other hospitals. As I made my way to the lab to get my blood drawn, I passed a stairway and a large glass window with a graphic of a patient in a hospital bed. Physicians, scientists, and other patients with heroic silhouettes and the prominent words *First in Human* spanned across the image. I'd later learn this was referencing a documentary about the NIH, *First in Human*, which I actually quite enjoyed later on. But at the time, as I walked through the doors, my stomach sank as my eyes fixed on the words *first in human*—a stark reminder that since this was a research hospital, many of us here were out of options, searching for hope and at the end of the line, trialing treatments on the bleeding edge of medicine that had never been tried in humans before. Some have referred to the NIH as the National Institutes of Hope instead of the National Institutes of Health, as this place and the promise of treatments found here offer just that: hope. But the *first in human* bit was a reminder of the risks that hope carried, making my stomach turn.

I finally made my way to the lab and checked in. As I took a seat, I gazed around the room and took note of the other patients waiting in the lobby. There were a handful of us, but I and one other patient were the only ones who didn't seem to be accompanied by someone else. Just like I'd see in the atrium, it appeared to be medical professionals sitting alongside them, carrying on casual conversation. From what I could gather, it looked like most of the staff were here to have research samples drawn, a theory I put together solely on the containers they carried with them. But others seemed like they were waiting for the patient to finish their labs before escorting them to an appointment. I watched as a patient in front of me was called back and someone sitting beside her in a white coat fired off a response: "Don't worry, I'll just wait here for you to come back."

I'd never seen a health care team waiting on patients like that before and wasn't quite sure what to think. But it wasn't something I would have much time to ponder, as the thought was interrupted by the speaker now calling my number. "A-7, please make your way to station eighteen," an automated voice instructed overhead. I stood up and made my way to the door, where I was directed back to a long row of cubicles that looked straight out of a corporate office building. This was such a stark contrast to any center I'd been to before. The unease and pit in my stomach continued to grow. *If this place doesn't look like a hospital, can it really operate like one?* I thought to myself as I made my way back seven cubicles on the left.

A man named Wesly with kind eyes and a tattered lab coat greeted me. "Ms. Coleman?" he confirmed as he looked down at my wristband and gestured for me to sit. As I got settled, he scanned my band and began pulling different colored tubes from an organizer on the shelf, setting them in an area he had prepared beside me. "Looks like we've got quite a few today, huh, Ms. Coleman," he said, looking to connect as he rolled his chair over before catching the watery eyes I was trying to conceal. His eyes softened as he touched my arm gently with concern. "You okay, Ms. Coleman?"

"I'm okay. I'm just scared," I choked out, feeling overwhelmed.

"Are you scared of needles?" he gently asked.

"Yes," I replied, my heart racing and my breath quickening as I tried to ward off the panic attack I felt surfacing. "But it's not the needles," I confessed. "I have a big surgery coming up. I'm just scared and a bit overwhelmed. I'm sorry, I'll be okay." I said, ashamed and embarrassed by my inability to hold the emotions back.

"No, no, don't be sorry. I'll take good care of you, I promise," he said, gently tilting his head in an attempt to make eye contact despite the gaze I was shamefully casting toward the floor. "You'll be okay. I'm going to start, but if you don't feel good, you tell me, okay? But you're going to do great." He gave a gentle and encouraging pat as he leaned back to grab an alcohol swab to prep the vein. I looked over at the nearly twenty tubes sitting beside me, made a fist as instructed, and then closed my eyes.

"You're going to do great," he reassured me once again as I felt a small pinch. I kept my eyes closed, listening to the familiar pop of the rubber caps as one blood-filled tube was replaced by another. I appreciated Wesly's affirmations and check-ins every few draws, filling the space between. But as we reached the end of the stack, my hands began to feel clammy and my body grew warm. "I don't feel so great," I muttered softly.

He looked up with immediate concern, "You dizzy?"

"Yes," I confirmed, opening my eyes briefly before quickly closing them once more as the lightheadedness set in.

"You're going to be okay. I'm right here," he assured me as he swiftly filled the last tube, unhooked, and wrapped my arm before asking a passing phlebotomist to quickly grab a cold towel. He had me lean forward to rest my head on the desk while draping the towel across my neck, checking in with me every few seconds.

As a tear fell from the corner of my eye, I felt his concern deepen. Except this didn't feel like a medical response; it felt like an emotional one. His decades of health care training had kicked in to ease my symptoms, but I could see the emotional toll my fear seemed to have as he tried to comfort and console me.

In the weeks ahead and after a million trips down to that lab, Wesly would tell me I reminded him of his daughter. And when I asked about her, he'd proudly and adoringly share pictures of her and his grandkids. Suddenly, I recognized the emotion. It was the concern of a father.

Thankfully, after a few minutes, the lightheadedness began to fade. I apologized profusely, embarrassed that I couldn't handle something as simple as labs. But I knew this reaction wasn't about the needles or the tubes of blood stacked beside me. While they certainly didn't help, this was the manifestation of all the uncertainty and fear looming ahead and the frustration that I couldn't seem to get under control. I wished it were as simple as a fear of needles, something I could close my eyes and hide from, but there was no hiding or escaping these mounting fears that I knew would only continue to grow greater with each passing day until surgery.

As I gathered my things and attempted to stand up, Wes gestured for me to stay seated. "No, no, take your time. No rush. Sit here. I'll be back," he said, quickly popping out of the cubicle. He disappeared from sight briefly, only to return moments later with water and two apple juices in hand. "One for now, one for later," he explained as he handed them to me with a big smile spread across his face.

I graciously accepted the drinks, thanked him, and apologized once more. He shook his head as he helped me stand back up. "No need to be sorry," he reassured me. "Next time you come back, ask for me. I'll make sure you're okay."

I nodded with a smile as I left his cubicle. I felt grateful for his genuine care through a very vulnerable moment. I also felt a sense of guilt for my misconceptions and worry about the quality of care I'd receive based on the unconventional setup of the lab. While this facility was certainly different from the pristine and updated cancer centers I'd been to, my experience with Wesly served as a valuable lesson, teaching me that quality of care goes far beyond whoever has the latest gadgets, gizmos, or best branding—a reminder I'd have to continually adapt and learn from in the days ahead as I navigated from one lobby to another, meandering through a building that felt like an office filled with white lab coats and scrubs. Every experience or understanding I had of health care was about to be turned on its head.

24

NIH is currently low on O blood type donations and platelets needed for my surgery. If you live in the area and can donate at the NIH, it would truly mean the world to me and could help us proceed with surgery.
—Instagram post, June 6, 2021

A s I LEFT the lab behind, I opened my phone for directions to my next appointment and made my way to the nearest elevator bank in search of a directory or map without much luck. "Outpatient clinic three," I mumbled under my breath, looking to the elevator, my phone, and then down the hall again. *Where in the world is outpatient three?*

A young doctor approached, taking notice of my confusion while he called the elevator and awaited its arrival. "You lost?" he kindly asked.

"Yes, very," I replied. "I'm looking for outpatient clinic three."

"That's going to be on the third floor," he informed me. "I don't remember which end, but I can help you find it," he generously offered as the elevator arrived, gesturing for me to step in.

On the way up, he asked if it was my first time at the NIH. After I informed him that it was, he gave me the rundown on what I'd find on each floor, told me where the cafeteria was, and offered pointers on the best places and floors to escape to if I ever needed to find a quiet space. I was grateful for the mini tour and advice as we exited the elevators and made our way to a pair of double doors outside the clinic. "Just through there," he said as he sent me off with well wishes.

Everyone is so friendly here, I thought as I thanked him and reached for the door. On the other side, I found an empty room with a handful of chairs individually spaced six feet apart. There were also two long folding tables with suspended plastic shields, a couple of computers, and a printer at the end. They reminded me of the temporary registration tables I used to set up to check drivers in on race day. This didn't look like a clinic; maybe I was in the wrong place. A woman walked out from one of the rooms and asked if I needed to check in. Confused, I replied, "I don't know. I think I'm supposed to meet with hematology?"

"Hematology?" she repeated back. "Hematology is on the fifth floor."

I looked back down at my phone, confused. "They told me outpatient clinic three?"

"This is outpatient three, but hematology isn't this floor," she advised as she pointed me back to the elevators and instructed me on how to find the clinic.

On the fifth floor, I found myself going through the same song and dance. I walked through another set of double doors and was greeted by more folding tables with plexiglass shields and a handful of nurses waiting to help me get checked in. They asked for my doctor's name this time, but after confirming it, they advised me that she was planning to meet me at outpatient clinic three (OP3) and that I should head back downstairs. Thoroughly confused and turned around, I made my way back down to where I'd just come for one last try.

As I returned through the double doors, the nurse at the table greeted me once again. "You're back," she said. "Were you able to find the clinic?"

Overwhelmed and worried I might miss my appointment, I told her I'd found the clinic but they'd said I needed to come back down here.

Picking up on my distress, she quickly invited me over. "Let's check. What's your name, honey?"

I provided her my name, date of birth, and appointment time.

"There you are. When you said hematology, I pointed you upstairs, as I thought you were looking for their clinic. But it looks like you have appointments here this afternoon, so Dr. Kalsi will be coming to you. I'm sorry about that. Have a seat, and we'll get you all checked in. The doctor should be here shortly," she explained, both compassion and a hint of embarrassment about the miscommunication evident in her voice.

As I waited, I looked around at the empty room. I was wondering where all the patients were, confused about how everything felt so fluid and unorganized, when suddenly I heard a code blue called from the speaker overhead. I wasn't sure what exactly that was, but it sounded urgent, so I opened up my phone for a quick search to find that it meant "cardiac or respiratory arrest, medical emergency." This place felt so different from everything I was used to; I'd never heard a code blue—or any code, for that matter—called overhead before. My nerves and unease continued to grow.

I didn't know it at the time, but the NIH expected the best but meticulously planned for the worst to ensure they were never unprepared and their patients had the best outcomes possible. The code blues I heard when waiting for appointments, the several days planned in the ICU post surgery, and preparation plans for a catastrophic bleed were all part of their safety standards. Over time, I would come to realize that this experience was a combination of both unusual circumstances and some of the aspects I would grow to love most about the NIH. The very same experiences that were driving my unease would eventually be part of why I felt safer in their care than anywhere else.

I learned their threshold for code blues was much lower than at many other hospitals while getting an iron infusion later that day as another one sounded overhead. The nurse administering my infusion and keeping me company while it ran was one of the first to dart out of the room. When she returned, I asked in a concerned tone, "Does that happen a lot around here?"

"We're just extra cautious," she explained after reassuring me that the patient she'd just attended to would be completely fine and oftentimes a code blue here wouldn't be considered a code blue elsewhere. "Don't let that worry you, you're in good hands here," she kindly reassured me.

Even the empty waiting room and the confusion between appointments, I'd come to learn, was a by-product of the NIH's adaptive care. In order to bring me in and get everything sorted out with my bleeding disorder, they were shuffling everything around, and we weren't running on a normal schedule. Which explained why I found myself in an empty waiting room—it wasn't a normal clinic day. Also, in order to consolidate care, doctors often tracked patients down to meet wherever was most convenient, which was why Dr. Kalsi would be coming to me instead of me having to bounce from one clinic to another in search of her. The doctors here weren't stacked with forty patients to see every day, which gave them a flexibility to be present and extremely attentive. Lastly, those folding tables with the plexiglass shields would end up being temporary fixtures as well, for the construction they had underway. By next visit, I'd find a new nursing station in their place and a clinic that looked far more like a normal doctor's office.

It wasn't long before I was called back for vitals and to await Dr. Kalsi's arrival. The room was sterile, without any artwork or decor, but there was a computer in the corner with a screen saver shuffling through pictures of the hospital staff, offering a subtle sense of warmth and a distraction to pass the time. By the third loop, I heard a gentle knock at the door signaling Dr. Kalsi's arrival. She greeted me with a warm hello before pulling up a stool to take a seat.

As we ran through my history again briefly and the plans for further testing that week, I could feel the familiar sense of compassion that she'd shown during my first telehealth appointment. Despite the discomfort from all the blood draws and tests, I knew the pile of tubes that morning was a manifestation of her determination to ensure nothing slipped between the cracks. Due to the bleed that had occurred during my biopsy and my history of bleeding in the past, it was suspected that I had a bleeding disorder; we just didn't know which type yet. We were racing against the clock to diagnose it before surgery so we'd know how to treat it. There were still so many unknowns, but I felt safe and reassured in Dr. Kalsi's care.

Throughout the next few days, I had several more labs, scans, and appointments in preparation for surgery. And each evening I returned back to the hotel, exhausted and wishing Brian were there as I awaited the results. The pressure was mounting, and with everyone I knew and loved halfway across the country, I'd never felt so alone. I'd lie in bed each night, staring at the ceiling, wondering if I'd made a mistake as all the labels I'd been given over the past six months rang in my ears: "You're so strong, so brave, you're an inspiration." This certainly didn't feel like strength—it felt like survival.

When Wednesday rolled around, it was finally time to head home, but Bruce insisted that I needed a quick tour of the city first. He arrived at the NIH in the GTR, ready to be my chauffeur. I climbed in the passenger seat and buckled into the five-point harness, trying to remember the sequence for clipping in. The last time I'd found myself in a seat like this, I'd been doing hot laps around a racetrack at 105 miles an hour with a driver who seemed intent on marrying our car with the bumper ahead of us. There couldn't have been a greater contrast between that and Bruce, who very evidently was used to carting patients with cancer around. As we hit the road, he apologized for the rough ride and checked to ensure that none of the bumps or turns caused any pain before finally laying into the accelerator. I rolled down the window as we picked up speed to feel the wind on my face and hear the roar of the engine as we made our way across town. We'd take the long way to the airport, crossing over the Potomac River into DC and making a quick pit stop to check out the Lincoln Memorial and Washington Monument before my departure—a nice way to round out the trip with memories of something other than cancer.

I'd arrive back home a day before my mom flew in for a quick visit before surgery. Our relationship had become strained during the pandemic, something we'd tried to set aside, both recognizing the rising stakes of the surgery ahead. Our visit was brief, but I appreciated her company and found myself missing the close relationship we'd once shared. As we sat around the kitchen table playing games, I found myself hoping that on the other side of this surgery, we could find our way back to the closeness we'd lost. In the meantime, I was just grateful she was here and for the support she'd given us. The next day, Baxter would board a flight with her back to Utah and Brian and I would hit the road with Dora in tow, bound for Maryland.

Yes, we brought Dora, our cat, cross-country to Maryland to live with us in a hotel for a month. We knew both surgery and recovery were going to be taxing not only on me but on Brian as well, and Dora was Brian's security blanket. The two of us had navigated our new marriage and the uncertainty of my diagnosis well so far, but that didn't look like the fairy tale it sounds like on paper. We'd navigated the rough waters together by playing to our strengths, acknowledging our weaknesses, and supporting each other through the highs and lows. Brian was loyal and unwavering in his support, but pivoting was not his forte, and when things didn't go according to plan, he'd shut down. I could empathize with his frustrations in these moments, because I used to be the same way, but over the years, pivoting had become one of my strengths.

While I'd learned how to pivot, decision-making was not my strong suit, which was where Brian would step in for me—a statement that feels a bit ironic and unintuitive to people who know me post diagnosis, given the fact that I was forced to make so many life-changing decisions so quickly. But these decisions never came easily and took a lot to accomplish. My natural tendencies would often lead me into analysis paralysis for weeks when making even the smallest of decisions, and I would spiral until I became too overwhelmed to make any decision at all. Brian, on the other hand, just wanted a path to commit to, which meant he was good at pulling the trigger. Whenever I shut down because I was too overwhelmed by the thought of making a decision, he'd make it for us. Then, when he shut down because there were too many unknowns or external factors, I'd step in and execute. Our strengths and weaknesses played well to each other, but heading into surgery, we both knew all the uncertainty we were navigating was going to be more my forte than his. Except with me fresh out of surgery, I wasn't going to be of much help for at least a month. So insert Dora, who'd been Brian's one constant through any uncertainty he'd navigated over the past seven years. We'd bring her with us both as one less thing he'd have to worry about while we were away and as a sense of comfort and security in weathering the storm.

We originally planned on flying back to Maryland together. However, the reduction of COVID restrictions had led to a rush of summer travelers and a shortage of rental cars. After seeing the nearly $5,000 price tag that a rental was going to cost us for our stay, we decided to road trip it instead. Over the next few days, we'd take turns playing cat wrangler on the twenty-five-hour road trip until finally making it to the hotel that we'd call home for the next month.

We arrived late in the evening and checked into the hotel in the heart of downtown Bethesda, relieved to finally be off the road. We'd lost the entire weekend on the drive, and I had more lab work queued up for Monday morning, which was rapidly approaching. So we hauled Dora up to the room with us and quickly unpacked the essentials before lying down and attempting to catch some sleep for an early morning the following day. We were blissfully unaware of the nearly insurmountable obstacles we faced ahead.

The next morning, Brian dropped me off for labs—another stick and twelve more tubes in search of answers. There were still a few specialized tests pending from the week prior, but all the others we'd run had come back normal, which meant we weren't any closer to finding what type of bleeding disorder I had. It was crucial that we find out to ensure we could properly treat it for surgery. In an attempt to distract ourselves from the news and with a clear schedule for the rest of the afternoon, Brian and I decided to head down to the National Mall. This way he could get some sightseeing in too, since he hadn't ever been to DC.

We strolled along the same paths Bruce and I had the week prior, taking in the monuments and enjoying each other's company as I regurgitated the walking tour Bruce had given me as if I were an expert. I even was able to convince Brian to take a selfie or two with me to document our outing, like we were true tourists. For a moment, we felt like just another couple on vacation. Seeing us lost in the crowd and sea of people, you'd never be able to separate our lives from theirs. Unfortunately, that feeling would be fleeting. As my phone began to buzz, I looked down to see a call from the NIH.

I answered to find the PA from my team on the other end of the line. She gave me updates about the scans and tests planned for the following day, but she also let me know that since they hadn't been able to pinpoint my bleeding disorder yet, they'd encountered a bit of a hiccup. With my surgery being on both my kidney and liver, two hypervascular organs with the potential for high blood loss, they'd need at least sixty units of blood for my surgery alone and one hundred total on hand for the hospital. Due to the national blood shortage, the blood bank had only around thirty. If they weren't able to bring in the rest by the time of surgery, we'd be forced to reschedule with no guarantee of when or if they'd have enough at a later date.

Her voice was calm and collected. I could tell she was trying not to alarm me, but I was crushed. After all we'd been through over the past few months, was it all for nothing? I'd stopped treatment, upended our entire lives, and we'd just driven twenty-five hours cross-country after putting all our eggs in this basket, which had now spilled all over the floor. I tried to hold back the tears as I felt the hope drain from inside me, wondering if I'd just made the biggest mistake of my life. I asked if there was anything we could do and if we could help drive in donations. She informed me that if we knew anyone in the area that could donate, it would help close the gap, but they were doing everything they could on their end as well and she would keep me updated as the week progressed.

As soon as we hung up, Brian, who'd been listening in the distance concerned, asked for an update. My voice cracked as I desperately tried to hold it together, not wanting to break down in public while I broke the news about the blood shortage and the possibility of surgery being rescheduled.

"And they couldn't have told us before we drove all the way up here?" I could hear the frustration lacing his voice. It was a manifestation of all the stress and anticipation he'd been suppressing along with the helplessness of feeling like there was nothing he could do. He'd been skeptical of us coming to the NIH in the first place and of the pivot in plans after I'd already established care with Dr. Msaouel at MD Anderson. He was trying to be supportive, but the man who was notoriously bad at hiding his facial expressions had *I told you so* written all over his face. "So now what? We go back home?" he asked, his tone rich with resignation. It didn't matter that the surgery hadn't been rescheduled yet; we were thousands of miles from home, and in his mind, there was no way we could drive in the blood donations we needed. With the change in plans, I knew he was now shutting down. However, us both spiraling surely wouldn't get us anywhere, so this was my cue to step in. Time to pivot.

I tried to come up with solutions as we made our way back to the car. I had a stepbrother who lived in the area. I had no idea what blood type he was, and although I'd always looked up to him in many ways, we hadn't ever been particularly close. The only other person we knew in the area was Bruce. I could ask both of them, but I knew that wouldn't be enough. However, I wasn't willing to go down without a fight. So as a last-ditch effort as we climbed in the car and made our way back to the hotel, I edited one of the pictures we'd just taken together, overlooking the Washington Monument. In bold text I overlayed the words BLOOD DONATIONS NEEDED in the DC AREA for surgery next week on the photo and wrote out a long caption explaining our situation before hitting send and posting to both Facebook and Instagram. As I reread the post out loud to Brian, a wave of embarrassment washed over me. Was I really asking strangers for blood? I felt like a charity case. Instantly, I regretted my decision to post the request and asked him if I should take it down before realizing that unfortunately, at this very moment, I was a charity case. And quite honestly, we needed any help we could get. I'd have to swallow my pride, leave the post up, and hope for the best.

— 25 —

I believe the measure of an individual is not found in how
they handle the easy things in life, but rather the challenges.
It's clear you are in this world for all the right reasons.
—Jon Gerson, blood donor

WHEN I POSTED the call for donations, I didn't expect much of a response. I didn't have a large social media following at the time, mostly just my friends and family back home who'd been following along since my diagnosis. They'd all be too far away to help. However, after Bruce gave my post a little boost, it didn't take long before the notifications started pouring in, and by the next morning, my in-box was full with messages from countless strangers eager to help.

The outpouring of support continued to filter in as friends and family kept sharing and spreading the word. I hadn't had a chance to notify anyone at work, but after a coworker saw the post, they all began rallying around the cause. My boss ended up reaching out, offering to send out an email blast to the motorsport organizers and enthusiasts in the area. My long-time coworker and dear friend Ann helped get in touch with the blood bank to track the donations. She'd even go above and beyond, making an eight-hour drive to donate platelets herself in the coming days. I'd never in a million years expected to be met with this level of support. To be honest, as much as I wanted to live, I'd felt guilty about the ask. I didn't have kids or a legacy to leave behind and I didn't have much I could offer in return, yet here was a sea of strangers offering up far beyond just their sympathies, chipping in to give their literal blood for someone they'd never met.

The days that followed were a mixture of overwhelming gratitude and increasing fear. As the response to our plea for blood donations continued to pour in, I felt humbled and grateful beyond words. But with each appointment, it felt like the stakes were continuing to rise.

A few weeks prior, when we'd been given the green light for surgery, we'd been informed that the kidney portion would be relatively straightforward and that most of the risk and course of recovery would be driven by the liver. So when we'd met with Dr. Hernandez, the surgeon who would be operating on my liver a week later, I'd peppered him with a million questions, trying to understand the risks and just how big of a surgery this would be. While he acknowledged that it would technically be high risk, he didn't think that meant a high risk of death, which was what all my questions kept circling back to. In fact, he seemed pretty at ease about the whole thing. While my surgery was not simple, he had experience with others that had been far more complex. And since my tumors were very symmetrical and encapsulated, he wouldn't have to take very much of my actual liver, leaving me with plenty of function. While there were no guarantees and this was still a complex surgery, he confidently reassured us that he thought I'd do well and he wasn't too worried. We'd left that call feeling encouraged that maybe this wouldn't be nearly as bad as we'd been expecting.

However, now that we were on-site, I was starting to get a bit of a different impression. Over the next week, I met with numerous doctors and specialties in preparation for the big day. Each of them highlighted the unusual complexity of my case. I didn't leave a single appointment without someone mentioning how many times they'd been meeting as a group to discuss and prepare. Many pointed out that they'd met more about my case than they had for just about any other case before. I knew that, sensing my anxiety and anticipation, they were sharing this to provide me with reassurance that they'd planned out and accounted for every possible scenario to keep me safe. Unfortunately, it had the opposite effect. Instead of feeling reassured, I couldn't shake the growing sense that this was going to be much larger than I had anticipated. With each new conversation, I began to question my decision and wondered if my new team had the experience to pull this off. I was grateful that they were so carefully planning and preparing, but I'd gone from feeling like this surgery might be relatively small on the scale of procedures they'd do to feeling like I was one of the largest cases, requiring more coordination between departments than anything else they'd see all year.

As we drew closer to the end of the week, my nerves continued to mount. Navigating the corridors of the hospital from one appointment to another, I heard a periodic announcement emphasizing the urgent need for type O blood from June 15 through 29 and encouraging donations. There were also signs out at various locations around the hospital and in front of the phlebotomy lab. The first time I'd seen them had been before I knew about the shortage, and I remembered looking at the date and thinking what an odd coincidence it was that their drive ended the day of my surgery. But now that I realized they were likely at least in part for me, I'd walk by each one humbled by the efforts in motion but also reminded of the rising stakes. As I sat in phlebotomy for yet another round of labs, I stared at the sign ahead, replaying every conversation from the week.

I'd sent a text to one of the hematology fellows, Dr. Bryer, who'd been assigned to my case. Over the past week, many of the doctors and PAs I'd worked with had given me their cell phone number for direct communication. Which, I had to admit, was one of my favorite parts of the NIH so far; not having to go through MyChart or another health portal to send a message that took a minimum of a day to be triaged was refreshing. It felt a hundred times more efficient to contact my providers directly, as we were able to coordinate appointment changes, labs, and meeting locations on the fly.

Dr. Bryer had been helping to coordinate my care. She had a quiet confidence and an approachability that made me feel at ease. We were relatively close in age, which made her a comforting presence, and I often felt safe confiding in her. She'd checked in on me the night before, and I'd shared with her that I was uneasy and struggling with the number of mounting unknowns. So she'd asked me to notify her when I made it back to the NIH the following morning to touch base.

After one of my final blood draws, Dr. Bryer was waiting for me and greeted me outside the lab, and we made small talk as we made our way to a quiet room to further discuss my next steps with one of the attending doctors from hematology. Most of my testing had come back at this point, and I was looking for updates and answers to alleviate my concerns. I knew the greatest risk in my surgery was the risk of bleeding. Depending on what type of bleeding disorder I had, my team might be able to treat it and help mitigate some of the risks, which was why we'd be on a mad dash for such an extensive workup.

The hematology team was fairly certain they'd tracked down my bleeding disorder: von Willebrand disease, type 1. But they couldn't say this with any degree of certainty, as some tests were still pending. And while I'd had a response to a medication we'd tried the day prior, they didn't think it'd be sufficient to sustain me for the operation. So they'd ordered another medication that I should have a better response to. "Could," "should," "we think"—Dr. Bryer's language was laced with uncertainty as I pressed for answers. But there were some questions we just simply wouldn't have the answers for until I went under the knife.

Being a naturally analytical person, I struggled with this uncertainty. I wanted answers, I wanted statistics, I wanted to know my odds. But the answers were elusive; we simply didn't know. The surgery was high risk, a descriptor that felt like a moving target. But it was also my only shot. There wouldn't be time to reschedule and wait for more certainly. It was now or never.

I sat quietly for a moment, looking around the room, taking in the immense gravity of the situation I found myself in. I apologized in a defeated tone for all the questions I'd been asking, realizing that no matter how many times I asked, there were no new answers to be uncovered. "I just don't want to make a mistake," I admitted. "Without all the answers, I don't know how to make a decision. I don't know if I want to take the risk on Tuesday, knowing I may not wake back up, or if I'd rather let the disease run its course . . . enjoying whatever time I may have left." I trailed off, knowing I was asking a question they couldn't answer for me, as the decision ultimately rested on my shoulders. One that at thirty years old felt unfair and too heavy to bear.

I still had two more appointments before the end of the day, and all I wanted to do was head back to the hotel and escape from it all. But as the speakers overhead rang out with another announcement for donations, I pulled my phone from my pocket to see a long list of notifications. A rush of guilt washed over me. Here I was, questioning if I was even going to go through with the surgery, while selfless strangers were literally giving their blood to ensure it could happen. Even Brian would be heading over to the blood bank to donate later that afternoon. Over the past seventy-two hours, they'd become so inundated with donations that they'd extended their hours and were opening on the weekend in order to add more appointments. One of the employees who worked there informed me they hadn't seen this level of response in over fifteen years.

I opened my phone to respond to a few of the unread messages as I waited for my next appointment. There was a tagged Instagram story from a friend from high school whose sister was at the NIH, her arms wrapped in Coband, wishing me good luck. I saw a message from a former coworker who I'd learned had moved to the area and was offering to donate with her husband. Countless other messages had come in from strangers sending well wishes after donating, including a gentleman who despite being afraid of needles had just returned from his appointment and wrote that if I could face my fears, he could too.

How could I be questioning everything when each of these incredible humans had never stopped to question if they should help? It was far more than blood they were giving; they were providing me with a drive to push forward, one I'd take with me as I paged the elevator and tried to summon up the courage to make it through the next appointment without tears. My final scans were complete, and now that we had at least a vague idea of what my bleeding disorder might be and how we planned to treat it, I wanted to meet with Dr. Hernandez to check if everything was still on track.

I was generally aware of the number of tumors I had, even if it was a number that felt like it was constantly changing depending on who was reviewing and reading the scans. I knew the number specifically in my liver was a key factor in why I'd been turned down for surgery so many times before. In the ER, we'd been told there were likely four tumors; MD Anderson would tell us six; NIH had started with two, then it'd moved to four, and now, who knew. Part of the reason the number kept moving was because I hadn't had consistent imaging or a solid MRI yet. While I had gotten an MRI a few weeks after I was diagnosed, the image quality wasn't great, and the rest had been CT scans, which aren't nearly as sensitive as MRI for the liver.

In the lead-up to surgery, we continued to march ahead but always felt like we were treading on thin ice. I was constantly on edge, waiting for the rug to be pulled out from underneath us the moment they discovered additional tumors or found something they'd overlooked. I'd read study after study leading up to surgery about the criteria they used in both liver resections (cutting a section from your liver) and ablations (burning or freezing tumors) to determine if a procedure would be worth it. I'd been warned a hundred times about trying to interpret and apply other studies to my case, since what I had was so different. I knew the vast differences between cancers and even between subtypes of the same cancer. But with zero contextual knowledge to even get me in the right ballpark to ask questions, I was grasping at whatever I could get. The vast majority of these studies were pretty aligned on size and number of lesions being determining factors in eligibility for surgery. Although kidney cancer was not typically one of the types of cancer liver resections were considered for, I figured the likelihood of operating being a good idea or not might hinge on how many tumors they'd found in my liver. Which is what I wanted to discuss when I sat down in Dr. Hernandez's office.

I'd hoped Brian would be able to be with me for this appointment. Navigating all of these decisions on my own felt like an impossible task, and not having a second set of ears to confirm my understanding of everything made it even more difficult. But since he couldn't be there in person due to the COVID restrictions, I'd just have to patch him in on a call.

I tried to suppress my curiosity as I glanced around the room, taking in the various knickknacks, pictures, and books, trying to get a better sense of who the surgeon with a pompadour-style haircut and three-piece suit in front of me was. I'd always hated that the very people I was placing my life in the hands of were also the ones I knew the very least about. Each of them had a full summary and workup on me, yet all I seemed to know about them was their last name. A world where I know more about Susie, my neighbor from seven blocks over, through Facebook than I do about the doctors I entrust my life to had never sat right with me.

I didn't know much about Dr. Hernandez other than the fact that this was the second time I'd seen him in a three-piece suit. He had a stylish haircut, short on the sides and longer on top, that was combed back with a subtle wave. The salt-and-pepper specs peeking through suggested that he may be in his late thirties or early forties. He was impeccably dressed and exuded confidence.

"Hello, Miss Coleman, how are you today?" He greeted me in a friendly, casual tone, pushing back his chair from the computer to refocus his attention.

"Oh, I've been better," I said with nervous laughter at the basket case I'd been all day. He responded with a gentle laugh, fully aware of the anxiety and uncertainty I carried with me about the days ahead.

"Well, let's see what we can do about that. What questions do you have for me?" he asked as he leaned back confidently in his chair.

I patched Brian in on a call, and we dove into our questions. "After my scans resulted, were there any changes to my treatment plan? Do you still think you could get all of the tumors?" I asked.

He responded so swiftly that I briefly wondered if he had fully processed my question or if he'd had a full look at the scans. With the heightened emotional state I was in when I entered his office, this took me right back to the feelings I'd had leading up to my diagnosis, during a time when I'd often report symptoms to providers who already seemed convinced they were caused by anxiety before I finished speaking. It'd felt like they weren't genuinely listening or giving me a chance to be heard. As a result, I would often repeat myself or ask the questions in a slightly different way after any swift answers, just to ensure the answer remained unchanged.

I verified with him again, just to be sure. "So, you were able to see all the tumors in my liver?" I'd heard there were up to six, but originally I'd thought the NIH had only mentioned four. "Were you able to visualize them all?"

He nodded affirmatively, but his body language and tone left me pressing for more. It seemed as if he might have spotted more than six but was attempting to avoid alarming me, since it wouldn't alter the treatment plans.

"Were there more than six?" I hesitantly asked. I'd been off treatment for nearly a month and was worried about new growth.

"There might be a couple more. But I'm going to take care of anything that looks suspicious so we can get you to no evidence of disease. My goal is to leave you with no tumors behind," he assured me.

"A couple more?" I inquired further.

"A couple. I'm not worried," he confidently replied.

It was clear we were both beating around the bush. I suspected he knew a concrete number but didn't want to alarm me. And I was unsure if I really wanted to know how many there were if it wouldn't change our goals and we were still aiming at a surgery with curative intent. Which he confirmed.

Normally, vague answers are a surefire way to get me to spiral. Not understanding the rationale or all the variables at play will actually make me worry more than any potential bad news I may receive. I'd spent so long lost in the system that I felt like I needed to be hypervigilant to ensure it never happened again—planning out every worst-case scenario, knowing what to look for and the flags to raise before I ever found myself there. When I didn't have the full details or a clear picture, my mind would wander, thinking about all the things that could go wrong instead of focusing on the most likely outcome. Which would lead me into a never-ending rabbit hole. However, this time it was different. I knew I was at capacity and another ounce of bad news just might push me over the edge and get me to back out.

As I wrapped up my final questions and the appointment, I couldn't shake the feeling of doubt that had crept in. How could Dr. Hernandez be so confident when everyone else seemed to be more hesitant or concerned?

His confidence and quick answers retriggered memories of the past, which, through no fault of his own, added to my unease. But over time, I'd learn the confidence didn't stem from a lack of attention or preparation but instead his vast experience and expertise as not only a highly skilled surgeon but also a surgeon-scientist who ran an active lab at the NIH. His candor and straightforwardness would end up being one of my favorite parts of having him on my team, and something I greatly appreciate in him now as one of my most trusted doctors. But those weren't insights I had before going under the knife.

I found myself admittedly a bit lost trying to piece together the full picture of the risk ahead. Brian and I would have the weekend to think more about this before checking back in to the NIH Monday morning so I could be admitted for surgery the following day.

Until then, we explored Maryland. I knew I wanted to spend our last days before surgery visiting new places and making memories with Brian. Making the most of the time we had, just in case. But with all of the last-minute appointments and coordinating, I hadn't had time to plan the weekend for us. I wanted to take a drive to the coast at some point like we had in Houston, but I'd had no time to plan when and how.

While we both enjoyed taking drives together, I knew how frazzled Brian would get when we didn't have a set point or destination. I could drive for hours, just taking in my surroundings and letting the road lead wherever it might. But that wasn't exactly his jam. So by the time Saturday morning rolled around, I pulled up a map and looked for the first city on the coast with a name I recognized and claimed it for our route.

I sensed Brian's skepticism as we loaded into the car. "Why exactly are we going to Annapolis?" he asked with one eyebrow raised.

"To see the ocean," I replied confidently, hoping I'd get away with a vague answer and not give away my lack of planning. I mean, we were going to see the ocean. That part was definitely true.

"But where exactly are we going to see the ocean? Do you know where we're stopping?" he clarified, recalling the countless times I'd set us off on a drive with no planned destination and a few spontaneous wrong turns.

"Yeah, a park," I confirmed. That part was true too. When I'd pulled up maps, I had specifically found one along the water to map us to, but that was about as far as my plans had gone.

"And what are we going to do at the park?" he asked.

"Ocean stuff. It's a surprise, you'll see." A guilty smirk crept across my face.

While I had technically found a destination, we both knew I was winging the rest of this. He endearingly rolled his eyes and replied with a smirk back. "Ocean stuff, huh?"

"Yeah, you know, lots of fun oceany things. But I can't tell you because it's a surprise," I said as I put the car in drive and pulled out onto the main road.

"Right," he confirmed, shaking his head and adjusting the AC before leaning back and settling in for the ride.

About an hour later we arrived, pulling into a parking lot off to the side of the naval academy bridge that connected to a small park. It wasn't exactly the oceany things I'd been expecting. We didn't have a line of sight to an ounce of sand, and the park itself seemed a bit worn down. Broken benches, warped and rotted railings, and litter were scattered along the rocks. Brian looked over at me, less than amused as I smiled back and declared excitedly, "Look, the ocean!" trying to lift the mood as I reached for the door. I didn't have a plan. We both knew it, and I could tell Brian wasn't exactly happy about it.

As I closed the door behind me, I felt the emotion creep in and the facade of energy I had summoned quickly dissipate. I didn't care what our plans were for the day; I just wanted to do something, anything. This wasn't just an ordinary Saturday— the intrusive thoughts kept trying to convince me it might be my last Saturday. What if something went horribly wrong during surgery? What if they couldn't stop the bleeding, and what if I never woke up? I didn't want our last memories together to be passing time, flipping through channels on the hotel room TV. Yet, now that we were here, the idea of watching the waves crash in next to an empty bag of Cheetos and shards of shatter glass and forcing my grumpy husband to do "oceany things" didn't exactly seem ideal either.

I pulled it back together as I heard Brian approaching from the other side of the car, artificially inflating myself with energy to make sure we'd have a good time, but I couldn't hide the glossy eyes. Brian instantly knew something was wrong. And when he asked, I confessed that I didn't have a plan for today, that I just wanted to see the ocean and spend time with him. This wasn't quite what I'd been expecting; I could tell he didn't want to be here, and I felt like I'd ruined everything.

He admitted that being out in the hot sun wasn't exactly his idea of a good time but that if this was what I wanted to do, that's what he wanted to do. I felt both the hesitation and frustration in his voice. The man was trying to make me happy, but no part of this was enjoyable for him. He was trying, yet here I was, crying in the parking lot. I confessed to him how scared I was and how I desperately wanted us to have a good day together so that I could leave him with memories to remember me by. With a heavy heart, I looked down, kicking rocks at my feet as I mustered up the courage to admit the real reason I'd dragged us all the way across town. "I just don't want you to forget me . . ." My voice trailed off in a surge of tears.

Like a dagger to the chest, that one must have hit him as hard as it did me. I looked up to see his eyes fill before he surrounded me in a tight embrace.

"Nothing is going to happen. Everything is going to go great," he said as he leaned back to capture my gaze. "And I will never forget you," he vowed, tenderly wiping away a tear tracing a path down my cheek.

He hugged me tightly, and we both pulled it together before we continued on with our day's adventure. We strolled through the park until we finally came across a path leading out to the ocean and a cluster of large rocks, where we took a seat to watch the waves crash in. I leaned against Brian, tilting my head back and closing my eyes to feel the warmth of the sun on my face and listen to the soothing rhythm of the ocean. He draped his arm across my thigh and gently rested his head against mine, savoring the moment. I felt him pull back and kiss the top of my head and say, "So, is this oceany things?"

A smile spread across my face, "Yes, oceany things. Pretty great, huh?" I replied, my eyes still tightly closed, absorbing the serenity.

"Not too bad, I guess," he teased as he rested his head back against mine and we let the stress melt away.

We spent the rest of the weekend taking long walks shaded under the towering trees along Rock Creek trail and exploring our new surroundings before wrapping up with a visit to Bruce and Sarah's. Brian had never met or even spoken with Bruce, but instantly upon arrival he was surrounded by the same support they'd extended to me. In an unfamiliar city, as we faced the most extraordinary circumstances, they felt like family.

As we parted ways that evening, I thanked Bruce once more before quickly retreating down the front steps as I felt the emotions surfacing. This man had immeasurably changed my life—the connection to NIH, the blood drive, the dinners, the profound guidance. He'd taken me under his wing and had given us a gift I didn't know how I'd ever repay. I knew if I lingered even a second longer, I was going to turn into a puddle of tears. Bruce, humbly, never accepted the credit, but he knew how I felt.

I made my way out, laser focused on regaining my composure before reaching the bottom of the steps. I pivoted back around to wait for Brian, who was in the dimly lit doorway saying his goodbyes. I watched as a strong handshake morphed into a hug. Brian's eyes welled up with a mountain of gratitude as he paused and searched for the words to express his appreciation. But before he could find them, Bruce pulled him in for a hug, with two firm pats on the back conveying both an unspoken acknowledgement and steadfast support. Brian nodded his head as he made his exit. "Take care of her," Bruce advised as Brian made his way down the drive. "And good luck on Tuesday," he shouted to me as he stepped back inside and waved from behind the glass door gently swinging shut.

— 26 —

I know it probably feels like things are out of control right now, but just know that when you're SO close to your breakthrough, that's when negativity tries to knock you off of your feet. As hard as it is, stay positive and keep the faith. Love you Katie, and I can't wait to witness you kick cancers butt!!
—Message from MG, June 21, 2021

MONDAY MORNING, BRIAN and I packed my giant hospital duffel bag with everything we might need in the coming week and must-have recovery items suggested by other patients. It included a few pairs of oversized sweatpants I'd stolen from Brian, hoodies with wide arms that I could fit my IVs through, a phone charger long enough to wrap around the planet twice, ChapStick, and lots of card games to keep us busy. I was reaching down to make the final zip and lock in the bag's contents when I felt Dora brush against my leg, looking for attention. I plopped down on the floor next to her, giving her a few final chin rubs, promising we'd be back soon. Her familiar purr brought both comfort and guilt that we were leaving her behind.

While we were away, both Bruce and Alleigh, a nurse who'd helped take care of Andrew when he was undergoing treatment, were planning to check in on Dora for us. Brian and I hadn't had a chance to meet Alleigh yet, but we'd messaged back and forth on our way up, and after getting a sense of both her kindhearted nature and her love for cats, we knew Dora would be in good hands. Which we couldn't be more grateful for, as aside from the surgery itself, finding the right cat sitter was definitely Brian's greatest source of stress. We both felt relief in having someone we knew we could trust.

Before leaving, I did a final once-over on the room to see if we'd missed or forgotten anything. Out of the corner of my eye, I caught the gray hand-crocheted blanket draped over the side of the couch. It had arrived in a care package from my dear friend McKinley Grace a few days prior. Remembering how cold it had gotten last time I was in the hospital, I picked it up and squeezed it tight, trying to evaluate if it could help keep me warm. My fingers slipped through the holes as I pulled it close. It wasn't exactly made for warmth. If I brought it with me, it'd simply be for the support.

McKinley Grace, or MG, had been nineteen years old when she was diagnosed and when we'd met in one of the stage four support groups a few months ago. In the beginning, she was the only other patient I'd met who had an unclassified kidney cancer, which was the bucket mine fell into at the time as well—a classification that really just means "We're not quite sure what this is." Over time, she'd eventually end up being diagnosed with succinate dehydrogenase–deficient renal cell carcinoma (SDHB), a kidney cancer with under fifty metastatic cases reported, and I'd end up having a metastatic oncocytoma, one with under ten.

Over the few months before my surgery, we'd become a strong support system for each other, sending words of encouragement, exchanging messages from waiting room lobbies to ease the nerves, and offering a safe place to lay down our worries about the uncertainty ahead. This blanket was another manifestation of that. The blanket she'd given me was the first blanket she'd ever crocheted. With it had come a card full of encouragement and a small white decorative sign with the words *Yes You Can* embossed into it. I held the blanket close as I looked up at the sign, which I'd placed on the entertainment stand next to the TV. My stomach in knots from the nerves, I appreciated the symbolism and motivation.

I knew MG would have given anything to be in my shoes at that moment, yet here she was, sending me encouragement. I closed my eyes and let the words echo. *Yes You Can.* I then carefully folded the blanket, placing it back on the couch before throwing the strap of the bag over my shoulder. Looked like it'd be hospital blankets for me; this one was too valuable to risk losing.

After arriving at the NIH, we got approval for Brian to join me for my preop appointments, and we shuffled to and from the remaining appointments I had scheduled before surgery the next day. First up was internal medicine to evaluate if I had any red flags or major risk for surgery. Once receiving the all clear there, we met with anesthesia to go over consent.

At each appointment, the same conversations circled once again—discussions about how big a surgery this was, how often the team had met to review my case, and just how unique a situation this was. My confidence at that point was like a house of cards and each appointment added to the delicately balanced stack, ready to topple it at any minute. The minute we sat down with anesthesia, the wind began to blow.

The anesthesiologist was very attentive and compassionate as she took my history and began evaluating and disclosing the risks. She wanted to make sure she prepared us for the chance that I might still have a breathing tube placed when I woke up from surgery. I tried to quantify the risk, asking the likelihood of it happening. Surely this was just one of those "In case of emergency, you'll find a life vest under your seat" kind of warnings they gave everyone, right? I expected to hear the risk was very low but instead found the three haunting words that seemed to keep following me everywhere: "We don't know."

They had a pretty good hold on my bleeding disorder, but there was no way to know for sure, and we might not know until surgery. If they got into a situation where the risk of bleeding was too high for them to remove the tube, I might be woken up with it and not have it taken out until it was safe to do so.

My mind raced back to all of the horror stories I'd heard over the past year of people being intubated for COVID—the descriptions of patients experiencing confusion and discomfort and feeling like they were choking or suffocating. Was I really about to sign on a dotted line to willingly be woken back up like that?

We continued to discuss the risks of a long procedure—the risks from anesthesia itself and the things to look out for. I knew this surgery carried risks and knew it was their job to educate me about them. But what I didn't know was how in the world I was going to muster the strength to get through all this. With so many different ways things could go wrong, it seemed nearly impossible for anything to go right. I gave my consent anyway.

As we walked out of the office, I paused and gazed out the windows onto the vast NIH campus below. My eyes filled as I looked over to Brian. "I don't think I can do this." I felt my voice tremble and my leg begin to bounce.

"Yes, you can," he reassured me as he placed his hand on my back, gently swaying it back and forth in a show of support.

"No, I really don't think I can," I admitted, shifting my gaze back outside. "There are so many ways this can go wrong. No one has solid answers or confidence. No one can tell me what's going to happen. We're rolling the dice." I felt the frustration mounting and the tears making their way down my cheek. Except this time, the tears weren't fear based; it was frustration manifesting. I'd never felt so out of control in my entire life. I was faced with making by far the most important decision of either of our lives while flying completely blind. "I just don't know if it's worth it. If we can get another six months together, I don't want to throw that all away tomorrow. But that's the problem, NO ONE KNOWS!" I said as I broke down, leaning into Brian's embrace. "How am I supposed to know if I'm making a mistake if no one has answers?" I paused. "I'm not strong enough for this," I confessed.

Brian pulled me in close. "First of all, you are strong enough for this. You're the strongest person I know. Look where we are right now. You fought to get here. You can do this." His fingers gently ran through my hair. "But also, you don't have to do this. If you're not comfortable with it, this is your choice. You don't have to go through with it."

"I don't want it to be my choice. Plus they've had so many meetings, the blood drive, all the testing. I can't back out now; everyone will hate me. I will have wasted everyone's time and so many resources. I'm too far in, I can't turn back." I explained.

"Who cares what they think?" Brian argued, a protective frustration seeping into his voice. "This is your life, our life. I don't care what anyone else thinks. You need to be comfortable with this—" His impassioned speech was cut short by my phone vibrating against his back, as my arms were wrapped tightly around him. I pulled my phone back to see the number come across the screen. It was the PA who'd been helping us prepare for surgery and guiding me through my appointments.

Brian and I had gotten lost through the long, winding corridors of the hospital trying to find anesthesia earlier. The PA was calling to ensure we'd made it and also to let me know I needed one more set of labs drawn, then I should head back to the room to have an IV placed for tomorrow. Surgery would be at eight thirty the following morning, and even though visiting hours didn't start until nine, Brian could come early to see me before it was time to head back, she explained.

"Wait, Brian won't be able to stay with me overnight through surgery?" I had to reconfirm to ensure I'd heard her correctly. I felt the house of cards that was sheltering what was left of my fragile confidence begin to give way. Without Brian there, I certainly wouldn't have the strength to go through with the surgery. The fear was evident in my voice as I let the PA know this and asked if I could call her back in a bit after we'd had time to evaluate our decision. She agreed but, sensing our distress, also reassured me she'd get to work on her end to see what she could do.

As I got off the phone, I looked to Brian and shook my head with tears in my eyes, "I can't do it. We're not doing it." He hugged me tight and tried to stop my spiral, assuring me he'd never leave my side. Both defeated and utterly exhausted, I wanted to go home. But he convinced me to at least go through with the final set of labs and to head back to the room while we waited for more information. This was a shift in our dynamic. I was usually the one pushing us through the roadblocks, but I simply didn't have it in me this time. With no footing of my own, I needed his to stand on.

After a visit with Wesley and a very heartfelt interaction and encouragement from one of the experts they'd brought to run labs for my surgery, I felt my spirits rise as Brian and I made our way back to the room. Upon our arrival, my nurse informed us that Brian had been cleared to stay—the only stipulation was that if he did, he wouldn't be allowed to leave the building for the duration. Which felt like a minor inconvenience in comparison. We looked to each other with relief, a giant weight lifted off our shoulders. I immediately texted the PA to thank her.

Not long after we settled back into the room, there was a knock at the door, and in piled a parade of doctors. Dr. Hernandez entered the room first, followed by Dr. Ball, the surgeon who was operating on my kidney; hematology; and each of the fellows on my case. They'd decided to come together instead of individually to check in ahead of surgery and make sure I was comfortable going through with everything. As we chatted, I raised all the same questions and was met again with the same unknowns. While they believed they had narrowed down my bleeding disorder, we still wouldn't really know until they made the first cut. But they were prepared for that. They had enough blood in the blood bank on hand, and Dr. Hernandez was going to take a stepwise approach, making a small incision to go after one of the smallest tumors first to assess the bleeding before going after the rest. If he thought it was too severe, he'd stop and they'd close me up to prevent any further complications.

The idea of going through all of this and being stitched right back up with all my tumors intact sounded less than ideal, but it beat the alternative. I wanted a crystal ball, and I wanted concrete answers, but there were simply no definitive answers to give. After several rounds of questions, Dr. Hernandez, who'd taken a seat on the hospital bed across from me, stated bluntly, "At a certain point, you're going to have to decide if you trust in us enough to go through with the surgery. No one else can make that decision for you. It's up to you."

We'd all been beating around the bush over this for the past few weeks. I'd gone in circles asking a million questions, hoping the answers would help get me there. The truth was, I didn't want to make this decision. I didn't feel like I had enough information to make it, but I also knew I wouldn't be getting any more. Between that and the idea of trusting people I'd spent at best an hour total with to hold my life in their hands, it all felt so unnatural. But there was something about Dr. Hernandez calling it out that, oddly enough, did spark a flicker of trust. It felt like he was acknowledging that where I lacked answers, I was going to have to rely purely on trust. The question hit me head on: did I and could I trust them with my life? I took a second, looked around the room, and realized just how many doctors I had rallying around my case, all of them here to help see me through this. And while I didn't truly know a single one of them, it was time to let go and put my trust in them.

Every ounce of it felt unnatural. It had taken six months of questioning every opinion and every answer I'd received to even get to this moment. On top of that, I was carrying years of baggage with me from having been dismissed and misled for so long leading up to my diagnosis. That baggage was heavy and wasn't easy to set down. But even though we did not know the final destination, I recognized that I was now in a room full of outstretched hands, ready to lighten the load.

I agreed to the surgery, put my trust in their abilities, and I felt their collective desire to see me through it as they got up to leave. The next time I'd see them would be as they were wheeling me back into the OR the next morning. Or at least everyone other than Dr. Ball, who returned to check in one final time that evening, leaving us with an interaction I'd cherish and appreciate for years to come.

With a gentle knock at the door, in walked Dr. Ball with a soft red cooler tucked under his arm that I'd seen Brian return with after his blood donation last week. He greeted us as he entered, letting us know he was just heading out for the day but he wanted to stop by and check on me. He pulled up a chair and settled in.

He answered my questions with a quiet but confident ease that I found comforting. I remember being taken aback by how relaxed he appeared. Kicked back like an old friend stopping by to visit, he was unrushed and never made me feel like a burden on his time, which was striking for someone who in many regards was recognized as one of the top surgeons in the country in his field. At one point in the conversation, he stopped to ask how I was feeling. Thinking he meant clinically, I proceeded to tell him I felt okay—no pains or major complaints at the moment. He nodded his head, glad I clinically was feeling okay, but he paused and asked the question one more time, with more emphasis not just on how I was feeling but on how I was holding up.

The question stopped me in my tracks. I'd always been pretty miserable at hiding my nerves, but I made an effort to not directly mention my anxiety to a doctor whenever I could avoid it. I'd seen it used against me too many times before, since it was often used to dismiss or write off my symptoms based on the anxiety I presented them with.

I remembered that at one appointment, I'd specifically asked if my weight loss was happening at a normal pace or if it could be a sign of something more serious, "like cancer." In the same appointment, I'd mentioned having night sweats, thinning hair, and severe abdominal cramps. But in my after-visit summary, there was a note indicating that I'd denied having "fevers, night sweats or weight loss," which was certainly not the case. After that interaction, I'd learned that it was best to avoid mentioning how I was emotionally feeling in any clinical presentation if I could and to focus on the physical symptoms at hand.

However, I could tell by the tone of Dr. Ball's voice that this was different. I responded honestly, disclosing just how nervous and scared I was. I expected to be met with reasoning but instead found empathy. He sat back and nodded his head thoughtfully before validating my concerns and acknowledging how overwhelming it must feel to be facing so many unknowns. He could see why I was scared. While the team might not have all the answers, he said, he promised I was in good hands and they'd do everything they could to keep me safe.

Everyone had shared with me their preparations in an effort to provide comfort, but no one had directly acknowledged the difficulty of the decision I was forced to make. There was something about the acknowledgment of it on such a real, human-to-human level that really set a foundation of trust for me.

Over the past week, I'd been beating myself up, wishing I was stronger and feeling weak for being so scared, which in turn had only made me question everything and whether I really had what it took to go through with this thing. But Dr. Ball's acknowledgment felt oddly encouraging. Maybe I wasn't too weak for this. Maybe having cancer and everything I was facing was just really, really hard. Maybe it was normal to be scared.

Dr. Ball stayed to answer a few more questions and to chat with Brian and me a little longer before heading out with that little red cooler tucked under his arm. As he left the room, I turned to Brian and asked if he thought Dr. Ball had donated for my surgery—an ask that felt a bit silly and self-centered. Doctors didn't do that kind of thing, I thought—it was probably just a coincidence. I'd later find out that not only had he donated for my surgery, but so had Dr. Webster, the fellow on my case. Doctors may not normally do that sort of thing, but when you strip away the title, people do. I don't know if a gesture has ever meant more.

— 27 —

This wasn't quite what I meant when I said I wanted a oncocytoma.
—Instagram post, June 25, 2021

THE MORNING OF the surgery, I stood in front of the mirror, looking at a face that felt unrecognizable to me. As a result of the treatment I was on to keep the tumors at bay prior to surgery, my hair had lightened and the sparse eyebrows I'd once had were nearly completely invisible. Which, paired with my bloodshot eyes from a restless night, caught me off guard. To hide these side effects, I had been taking pictures cropping out the top of my head to hide my lightening roots coming in or throwing on a ball cap whenever I could. And I'd spent a little more time filling in my eyebrows each morning before starting my day. But after showering, taking off every ounce of makeup, and throwing on an oversized hospital gown, I had nothing left to hide behind.

I'd never really thought I "looked" like a cancer patient before, but this woman in front of me didn't look like me. I remember feeling my own vanity creeping in and the sadness I felt in wondering whether, if things went south, this would be how Brian would remember me: the no-eyebrowed stranger in the mirror.

I nervously climbed into the hospital bed to be wheeled back to the preop area, where they'd promised I'd get to see

Brian one more time before I went under. I could feel my heart racing in my chest as we made our way through the corridors of the hospital, unsure if my shivering was brought on by the nerves or the drop in temperature as we moved through the surgical wing.

After consenting and signing off for surgery, they brought Brian back one last time. I looked up at him; my vision blurred from the tears as he reached for my hand. "You've got this," he encouraged, squeezing tighter as he fought back the emotion in his voice. "I'm going to see you in a couple hours, okay? I love you so much." His voice cracked as I felt a tear slip down my face.

I slowly nodded my head, paralyzed with fear and at a loss for words as I looked up at him, wishing he could stay longer. Unfortunately, the nurse was already ushering him back out of the room. He leaned in for a final kiss, and as he began to step away before our hands parted, I squeezed three time. *I love you.* He instantly broke into tears. "I love you. I'm going to see you soon," he said as our hands parted and he followed the nurse out of the room.

For the next six hours he'd anxiously await updates on how surgery was going. The first update came after they'd made the first cut with minimal bleeding, allowing them to continue, and further updates came throughout the day. About halfway through, he received a text from Bruce, who showed up with lunch in hand to ensure he ate and to offer a distraction. Bruce invited Brian to join him and Brad, another patient who was at the NIH for treatment, to eat and chat in the lobby for a while to pass the time—one of the most meaningful meals he'd ever had—before he made his way back to the waiting room to await the final updates, which came from both Dr. Ball and Dr. Hernandez about six hours later. They let him know that surgery was complete and that, although there had been more tumors than they were expecting, around fifteen in total, they believed they had gotten them all.

He finally breathed a sigh of relief as he headed back to the ICU, patiently waiting at my bedside for me to wake up.

To this day, when I ask him what his happiest memory of our relationship is, he always replies with this moment. There was so much uncertainty leading up to that surgery, and the six hours I was under were near torture for him. The moment he heard that I'd not only made it through the surgery okay but also that the surgeons believed they'd gotten all the cancer was one he describes as one of the happiest of his life. After all the heartache and uncertainty, all the obstacles and set-backs, for the first time, there was hope. There was no longer a guaranteed heartbreak at the end of our love story—no more worrying about being both a newlywed and a widower. There was light at the end of the tunnel, and for the first time, he had permission to envision it.

My memory of this moment felt much less euphoric. I woke up feeling like I'd just been flattened by a freight train and confused by the marveled look in Brian's eyes. I'd made it out of the surgery alive, but I certainly didn't feel like I was out of the woods yet. I knew my greatest risk for a bleed was within the first few days after surgery, and I wasn't going to count my chickens until we made it through that window. With me being high as a kite and unable to keep my eyes open long, counting chickens would be an impossible task anyway. Instead, I squeezed Brian's hand three times, lay back, and tried to force myself to sleep through it.

Unfortunately, sleep would be a generous description for all the tossing and turning I'd do for the next several days—although technically I couldn't physically toss nor turn. I'd never imagined anything would be more stressful than the surgery itself, but the next few weeks would make any stress I'd felt up until that point feel like child's play.

I spent the first forty-eight hours of the recovery quiet and drawn inward, just trying to make it through the day. I didn't sleep a wink but kept my eyes shut, persistently trying to coax myself into sleep—which proved to be a futile effort between the constant stream of people in and out of the room and my ever-racing thoughts.

The pain was substantial, but I remember being surprised at how well it was managed, never surpassing a five or six on the pain scale. The pain itself wasn't what was keeping me from sleep; instead it was the endless procession of storming thoughts as I tried to stay hypervigilant for anything that could go wrong. My life experiences up until that point had taught me to expect the unexpected, and I felt the trauma of those experiences resurfacing while I waited out the recovery.

I finally felt like I might be turning a corner and could catch some sleep once I recovered enough to move from the ICU back to the main floor. But unfortunately, just as I thought I'd made it past the worst of it, I was respooked by a nurse from anesthesia who had major concerns about the central line—a very large IV that accessed the main artery going to my heart and was sticking out of my neck. He was surprised to see me back on the floor with it, since he believed the removal of the line carried a higher risk of a catastrophic bleed than my entire surgery did. This wasn't quite the case, but who was I to question his evaluation? I certainly didn't have any medical training. He stressed several times the importance of me not letting anyone touch it.

So for the next twenty-four hours until it was removed, I was hypervigilant about it and didn't sleep a wink, worried that I tossed or turned in the wrong way, I'd disturb it, causing a massive bleed. These fears were a bit irrational, but with my stress levels at a ten, I didn't have much to go off besides the stark warning I'd received earlier that day. Poor Brian was such a good sport, putting up with me constantly asking him to check on it to make sure it looked okay.

Due to the risk of a bleed, I'd need to go back to the ICU for the afternoon in order to have it taken out. They would remove the line in the ICU, and I'd stay for monitoring for a few hours before making my way back to my room on the floor that evening. That was the plan, at least, but unfortunately, my body missed the memo.

A transporter swung by to pick me up and take me back to the ICU by midafternoon. We made our way to an empty room at the end of the unit, where a young nurse was there to warmly greet us. She made small talk as she helped transfer me onto the bed, laid me back, and began prepping materials for the removal. I wasn't usually big on small talk before a procedure, but I found both her presence and conversation calming.

After prepping the area and materials, she checked in with me once more to ensure I was ready, and I made a final exhale before clenching my eyes closed and grabbing Brian's hand as I felt her snip the stitches at my neck holding the line in place.

"You're going to do great," she reassured me. "Now, hold your breath in three, two, one . . ." I felt a swift pull as the tube was extracted from my neck. "Perfect, go ahead and breathe normally now. I'm going to be here applying pressure for a while. You did great—now we just hang tight," she said, a congratulatory tone filling her voice as she passed along a gentle pat of approval.

All right, that didn't seem too bad, I thought to myself as I loosened the death grip I had on Brian's hand. Now all we needed to do was wait it out. Every few minutes, I'd feel the nurse shift her positioning for better leverage as she applied an unrelenting force against my neck, pausing at five minutes, ten minutes, then fifteen to check the status of the bleeding before the wound finally sealed off enough for her to dress it and leave it be.

The whole process felt very anticlimactic and wasn't anything like I'd been expecting. I began to question the warning from anesthesia about this being the riskiest part of surgery and felt embarrassment creep in over how worried about it I'd been. I thanked my nurse for her patience and joked about what a chicken I was, which she softly chucked at before reassuring me I'd done great as she tidied up the rest of the supplies. As she wrapped up, she passed along heartfelt wishes for a smooth recovery and a parting dose of uplifting encouragement before stepping out of the room.

The nurse who came in to take her place carried an air of frazzled urgency, bumping and pulling at my IVs as she adjusted the bed to prop me up. I could tell she had other patients to attend to, and I felt bad that I was probably an unexpected add-on to her shift for a few hours. But since removal of the line had gone well, hopefully we'd be heading back down to the floor soon.

As we waited, I felt the giant jug of water I'd been sipping on all afternoon catching up with me. Just a few hours prior to arriving in the ICU, we'd pulled the catheter that'd been in place the past few days, which meant I hadn't had to think about using the restroom until now—a seemingly daunting task, as my lack of mobility prevented me from sitting or standing on my own. I was hoping I could make it until we were transferred back down to the main floor. My favorite nurse, Kate, had been on shift, and I knew she'd be able to help navigate the incredibly awkward situation, knowing I was going to need help getting up and down. But as the urgency grew, I realized I didn't have a choice and notified my nurse the next time she stopped by.

I could tell she hadn't planned on a stop long enough to help me get to the restroom. I watched her pause and try to shift gears, recalculating how much time she had to get through her next task. She moved quickly as she set down her things to assist me out of bed, snagging and pinching my IVs again along the way. I sure missed Kate.

I shuffled my way over to the bathroom in the corner of the room. As I sat down, Brian wheeled the walker in front of me for added stability and for the assist when it came time to get backup. The nurse must have supposed he had it from there, because when the time came to make it back to the bed, she'd already stepped back out of the room. I thought she might be right back in, but after a few minutes, we realized we were probably on our own.

Brian had helped me out of bed several times at this point, an activity that reminded me of a Turkish get-up, my least favorite CrossFit maneuver. My process had evolved into a series of moves. First, I'd position an arm behind me to push up and lift my torso off the bed. Next, I'd drop my left leg off the side and use the momentum to reposition my arm for more leverage. From there I'd halfheartedly roll to the side and kick my other leg around. Once I was in a seated position, the bed was usually high enough that I could shimmy myself to the edge and use the walker to hold my weight until I got my footing under me to take care of the rest. I'd done this tango enough that I knew I could get out of bed. But unfortunately, in my current predicament, I found myself seated much lower without any leverage.

I counted to three as I gently swung my weight back, hoping the momentum would help lift me onto my feet. I hadn't even made it a quarter of the way up before I felt a sharp pain in my stomach and fell back down. "I think I'm stuck," I said to Brian in defeated embarrassment. I knew we needed help, but I was too embarrassed to ask and too worried about pulling my nurse away from much more mission-critical care. Keeping people alive felt far more important than lifting the woman at the end of the hall off the toilet because she wasn't strong enough to stand back up on her own.

Grasping for the only sense of dignity I felt I had left, I gave it one more try. "Three, two, one . . . ," I whispered under my breath as I leaned back and swung up one more time. I shifted the momentum into my legs as I lifted with twice the effort I'd applied before, and Brian steadied me with his arms under mine. The intense pain resurfaced, but I doubled down through it, knowing I was almost there. As I made it to the top, I locked my arms out on the walker to lighten the load as I tried to catch my breath. I felt frustrated that even the smallest efforts felt like Herculean feats.

With a short exhale, I let out a triumphant "Okay" with a mixture of pride and exhaustion. Mission accomplished. Now all I needed to do was make it back to the bed. I lifted my head and took one small step forward before I felt my face flush, my hands go clammy, and my vision fade. Uh-oh. I'd been through this song and dance before and knew exactly what was coming next. Knowing I didn't have much time, I quickly warned Brian, "Get help—you're going to need to get help!" as I tried to lower my center of gravity to reclaim the blood flow.

I heard the panic in his voice as he tried to process what was wrong.

"I know this feeling. I'm going down," I said, just as the pain disappeared and my vision faded to black.

Brian tried to catch me but only slowed my fall as I plummeted back, hitting my head against the unforgiving metal plumbing concealed behind the toilet. I was completely out, with no awareness of the passing time, while he desperately shouted and called out for help. As I was slumped over, each minute felt like an eternity for him until a nurse not assigned to my room came rushing in.

She hurried over and crouched down to assess the situation while Brian tried to relay to her what had happened, just as my memory faded back in.

I was surrounded by complete blackness as I heard their voices in the background. Brian's was laced with both fear and adrenaline as he helplessly looked on. And I could hear a woman's voice, concerned, as they tried to get me to wake up.

I knew I'd fallen. I could clearly remember the exact moment I'd gone down. But now, no one could seem to hear me. I knew the nurse and Brian were surrounding me, because

I could hear their bickering back and forth as the nurse tried to get Brian to calm down. I knew she was trying to assist me, but I couldn't feel her touch. I didn't realize I wasn't fully awake until I tried providing reassurance to Brian.

"No, I'm fine. I promise," I muttered, clearly without making a sound, as the commotion continued on without pause. I could hear him in the background, desperately trying to reiterate that I'd hit my head, trying to get the nurse to check it. "NO, REALLY—I'M OKAY! I PROMISE, THERE'S NO PAIN!" I said, trying to shout louder, something I thought they could hear even though no sound was actually coming out.

I paused for a moment, realizing what I'd just said. I knew I'd just had a massive surgery, but in this very moment, there wasn't an ounce of pain. It was as if my consciousness were peacefully floating behind a wall, without a care in the world, except for the mounting frustration that I couldn't communicate that I was fine or control the chaos unfolding on the other side. I heard Brian's voice becoming more animated as I gave it one more shot, this time feeling a rush as I opened my eyes to the bustling room. "I'm okay," I muttered with much less enthusiasm and oomph than I'd put into it a second before as I now felt a throbbing pain radiating from my abdomen.

I watched the relief spread across both their faces; it was clear they'd heard me this time. With an assist under each arm, they helped me to my feet and back over to the bed. Guess that was karma for labeling the central line pull anticlimactic. My body had decided to liven things up a bit. Lesson learned.

What I'd thought would be a quick trip up to the ICU ended up earning me another night there after the fall. It would also be the first and only time I've ever had to "fire" a nurse from my care. Which I felt terrible doing, but when the care didn't improve upon her return and after a couple more pulls on my IVs, we just needed someone else. This was the one and only time I've had less than ideal care while physically at the NIH. And to this day, I feel safer there for surgery than anywhere else.

After a fresh set of labs, despite the low-grade fever and chills I couldn't seem to shake, everything was still in decent shape, given the circumstances. My hemoglobin had dropped, requiring another blood transfusion, and my electrolytes were a bit out of whack, meaning I'd need a potassium infusion as well. The latter came with a burn that I can only describe as shooting your veins with lighter fluid and striking a match. The discomfort became so overwhelming that I backed out halfway through and opted for the giant horse pills to bring up my levels instead. But despite the rather eventful afternoon, I was grateful to have fared well and thankful to head back to a room on the main floor the following day for the rest of my stay.

— 28 —

*Over the past 2 weeks, through surgery, he never left my
side—not even once. Which meant sleeping on chairs
converted into beds and running on just a few hours of
sleep. I'll never know what I did to deserve love and a man
like this but my love for him is infinite.*

—Instagram post, July 11, 2021

WITH THE CENTRAL line removed and one more milestone down, I gave myself permission to switch from
survival to recovery mode. It wasn't a matter of whether I
made it out of the hospital—it was when. With a newfound
determination, I got dressed for the first time in days, carefully
stringing my IVs through the wide sleeves of my shirt and
stepping one foot, then the other, into Brian's oversized sweatpants, which he'd shimmy up my legs for me. My outfit was
complete with a ball cap to cover the rat's nest of hair sitting
on top of my head that hadn't been washed in days.

Each morning, one of the doctors would stop by on rounds,
grab a blue marker from the tray, and scribble a number on the
board, signifying the number of laps they wanted me to take
around the unit. My first goal would be sixteen laps, the equiva-
lent of one mile. This was a stretch goal that felt impossible at the
time, as I still was struggling to shuffle back and forth around
the room. But you can't give me a goal like that and expect me to
come up short. By the day's end, I was utterly exhausted, but when
the doctors came by for their final rounds, next to the *16* scribbled
on the board were now seventeen tallies for each lap completed.

With nothing else to do to pass the time, I made that little blue number my daily challenge, trying to beat my laps and my "high score" from the previous day. Like clockwork, every hour or two, Brian would slide over my walker, I'd cautiously make it to my feet, and we'd head out to the hall. The first day, I couldn't complete a single lap before heading back to the room, and I found myself frustrated as the seventy-year-old man down the hall, Bob, continually out-lapped me. Brian kept having to remind me that the man probably hadn't just had both his liver and kidney sliced and diced at the same time as he urged me to slow down. These little walks were tiring, and they hurt, but they were the one thing I looked forward to the most each day—the only piece of my recovery I could contribute to or control.

By the end of the week, each time we'd head out, we'd come back with six tallies to add to the board. And I'd gone from mentally competing with Bob to making friends with other patients on the unit as we made our laps together. Like Dave, who was on his third surgery at the NIH. We swapped stories about how different our care had been there in all the best ways, which to a fly on the wall must have been some pretty strange conversations to overhear. "Oh, Dr. Ball cut into you too, huh? What a great guy, am I right?" The unexpected camaraderie found in those hallway laps was oddly comforting and made the days feel a little less lonely.

While our eight-day stay at the NIH felt like an eternity at times, it was filled with many silver linings—everything from Dr. Linehan coming down to visit and staying for nearly an hour, teaching me—when he'd caught on to my interest—not only about my disease but their learnings and findings from other kidney cancers over the years, to my nurse on the Fourth of July, who took us on an adventure through the abandoned halls of the hospital and up to the top floor so we could watch the fireworks light the night sky over downtown Bethesda. It was the fresh blueberries from the farmers' market that Bruce dropped off and the nurses cheering me on as they watched my progress unfold. I spent most of my days through recovery lost in a sea of worry, fears, and anxiety, but these silver linings made me feel normal and gave me something to look forward to each day. By the time discharge finally arrived, I was both excited to finally be leaving the hospital and also a little uneasy about the road ahead we now faced alone.

Although we were leaving the hospital, it wouldn't be to make our way back to Austin. For the next three weeks, Brian and I would be staying in Bethesda to ensure we were nearby for any potential late complications. Which meant home for the next three weeks would be the four-hundred-square-foot hotel room that Dora had been diligently guarding for us while we were away. Unsure of the shape the room would be in upon our arrival after our cat had been given free rein for a week, we were relieved when we opened the door to find Dora happy as a clam, flopped over on the couch, welcoming us home.

The next three weeks would be filled with a whirlwind of such stress and chaos that they now serve as a regular punch line for Brian and me anytime we revisit the memories. How that man put up with me in that tiny room for so long is still a mystery to me. Each day was a chaotic clone of the last, with everything and nothing happening all at the same time.

I'd start each morning with a groan as I practiced my Turkish get-up, trying to lift myself out of bed. After rising, I'd shuffle my way over to the pills on top of the dresser, tossing back a blood thinner and a Tylenol before making my way to the bathroom, where I'd gingerly lift my shirt to expose my stomach and eye the hockey stick–shaped incision etched across it. Despite promising myself that I wouldn't subject Brian to another viewing, I'd inevitably always give in, beckoning him in with a concerned "Is it supposed to look like that?" or a nervous declaration of "It's opening!" at the slightest change. I'd never imagined the first year of our marriage would be Brian examining my wounds, dressing oozing drains, and washing me down in the shower while I worked to regain my mobility.

After showering, it was time for breakfast. One egg, a handful of spinach, and a side of fruit fueled me up for the pacing I'd do around the room and down the hall the rest of the day. My labs showed values associated with clotting that were quite a bit higher than baseline for a normal person, so my biggest fear was developing a blood clot, since that was how my grandmother had passed while recovering from surgery just before Brian and I met. So while we'd been nervous about excessive bleeding leading up to surgery, I was now hyper-vigilant, worried about blood clots instead. Honestly, a little comically so. I never sat for over an hour or two. I would walk in circles around the perimeter of the room, carefully stepping over the clothes strewn across the floor, ensuring I got my eight thousand steps in every day—an arbitrary number I'd come up with after hearing from another patient who'd thrown a clot after four thousand a day. Surely doubling that would keep me in the clear.

I became so obsessed and consumed with the fear of throwing a clot that I'd even set an alarm to wake myself up every three to four hours each night so I could get up and pace around in the bathroom—which, in retrospect, is quite hilarious to admit. I knew how ridiculous this was at the time, which is why I did my pacing in the bathroom, hoping Brian wouldn't catch me and call me out. But I was so consumed by the fear that I didn't even have a toe still rooted in reality, and almost compulsively, like a ritual, I had to complete my steps.

If it wasn't the fear of a clot plaguing me, it was the fever I was sure was going to take me instead. I hadn't been sure I was going to make it through surgery, so after I did, I was terrified a minor oversight would steal the future that was finally coming back into view. Every afternoon, like clockwork, my temperature would begin rising: 99.5, 99.9, 100.1, 100.2 . . . always just under the threshold I'd been instructed to call in for, which left me constantly on edge. I'd wake each night, cold and shivering from the night sweats, and make a midnight swap-out of my towels. I swear I practically lived with a thermometer under my tongue for a month, and I can still hear Brian's slightly exasperated but always patient reassurance echoing in the background—"No . . . you don't have a fever"—as he rolled his eyes for the tenth time that day.

These memories and the absurdity of the stress we were both under at the time bring a good laugh to us now. But in the moment, the stress was relentless, like a marathon with no finish line in sight. When the end of the month rolled around, marking my final appointments and restaging scans, we were both ready to head back home, blissfully unaware that the fight wasn't quite over yet.

Sometimes it's hard to be "strong" when [bad] news comes
in. But today I'm grateful to be here, to be healing and
I'll let the news be hard today. Today sucks but hopefully
tomorrow will be better.
—Instagram post, July 30, 2021

I WENT FOR RESTAGING scans at the NIH, and we flew back home to await the results in the coming days. The surgery was aimed with curative intent, and even though by the time my surgeons had gotten in there they'd found over fifteen tumors, they'd burned or removed them and they were confident they'd gotten it all. So we were hopeful that when the call finally came, we'd be hearing the words "no evidence of disease" (NED) for the very first time—a destination that, when I was originally diagnosed, I had been told not to get too invested in, as it wasn't the goal of treatment. While the term *remission* isn't often used in the world of kidney cancer, you'll typically hear a similar disease state described as "no evidence of disease." While it doesn't mean "cured," it does mean you've reached a point where there is no detectable cancer found. It's the goal nearly every patient dreams of reaching. Since early in my diagnosis, I'd accepted that due to the extent of my disease, it'd be a state I'd likely never reach, but for the first time, it was actually in the realm of possibility. My stomach turned for days in anticipation.

I didn't have a formal appointment scheduled, but my surgeon was going to give me a call that Friday with the results.

I woke up early, turned on my ringer, and stayed glued to my phone the entire day. Like an antsy child on a road trip, I kept checking in with Dr. Hernandez's nurse, Cathleen, every hour or two. "Do we have a time yet?" "What about now, still on for this afternoon?" I was trying to play it cool, but I was failing miserably, the desperation, I'm sure, seeping through every message.

By midafternoon, their clinic was running behind, and it was clear my surgeon wouldn't be able to fit me in by the end of the day, so after a quick review, Cathleen called to give me the high-level update. She knew my scans would post over the weekend, and she didn't want me to be caught off guard or worried by the results. I braced myself and took a seat on the couch.

I felt nauseous, and the pit in my stomach grew as she delivered the update. Overall, they were satisfied with my scans, they thought everything looked great, but there were a few new spots the radiologist had called out in the report. Since we'd scanned so soon after surgery, just one month out, there was no telling what exactly they were. It was possible they could be artifacts from surgery, so they weren't overly concerned. We'd rescan in a few months and follow their development. I felt the devastation wash over me as I tried to hold it together, trying to grasp and confirm the results.

I'd always known this was a possibility. The chance of new tumors popping up while I was recovering from surgery was why so many surgeons and institutions had turned me down before. But multiple new spots within a month would be a signal of aggressive disease. I repeated the words back for confirmation. "New spots; they said they're seeing several new spots?" The concern was clear in my voice.

She confirmed, adding clarifying context: the radiologists had to look extra closely and report anything that could be slightly concerning, but after reviewing my scans earlier that day, Dr. Hernandez wasn't too concerned. Although we didn't know exactly what the spots were, they were all very small, so he advised that we rescan in a few months after my body had more time to heal.

None of the "we're not concerned" bits were sticking, and all I could think about or hear was the fact that we'd found new lesions. This was supposed to be a celebratory call, the one where I expected to hear I was cancer-free, but instead, I hung up completely and utterly crushed.

I knew she'd called to provide reassurance and to save me from a weekend of distress, but I was still torturing myself over the results. I could hear the concern in her voice as she tried to prevent it, but I was already spiraling, and there was no coming back up for air.

I ended the call, and my head dropped into my hands and a puddle of tears began collecting inside them. Hearing my sobs down the hall and the subsequent pain they induced as I tried to catch my breath, Brian came in to check on me. He took a seat next to me on the couch, placing his hand on my back as he waited for the update that I physically couldn't get out. Since surgery, I had been unable to take a deep breath or completely fill my lungs without pain. As the heartache consumed me, I was left gasping for air.

We sat in silence as his hand swayed across my back, comforting me until I got everything back under control.

"It's back. There are three new spots," I said as the tears streamed down my face. "Three new spots in a month." My eyes hollowed with fear, refilled with tears. "Did we make a mistake? I can't go back on treatment . . ." My voice trailed off in exhaustion. "I don't want to go through that again. If it's this aggressive, I think I just want to enjoy the time we have." I looked up, and we locked eyes as I watched the words hit him like a cannonball to the chest.

"I think you may be jumping to conclusions here. Let's not get ahead of ourselves. Have you talked to Dr. Hernandez yet?" he asked, trying to reel me back in.

"No. But three new spots in a month. I don't know what else that could possibly mean. That's aggressive," I replied. "I don't think I'm strong enough to go through it all again," I said, closing my tear-soaked eyes and taking small, intentional breaths, trying to ward off both the mental and physical pain that statement triggered.

He kissed my forehead and rested his head against mine. "I still think we need to talk to your doctors, but I'll support you in whatever you decide." I felt the cold splash of his tears against my hairline as I squeezed his hand tightly, and I held my breath, trying to push myself through the emotional pain.

"I love you so much. I'm not making any decisions yet. I just think I need some time and space to process it all," I said as I looked up at him, kissing him back gently on the forehead before pressing my head to his as the tears fell between us.

At a zoomed-out view, I knew I was spiraling. The reminder that they weren't worried echoed in my head, but my mind wouldn't allow me to believe it. Flashing back to the day I was diagnosed in the ER, I recalled the words of the doctor who'd stepped into our room briefly after the ultrasound before they sent me for a CT: "We see a few things in your liver, but we're not too worried about it. We're going to get a better look."

They knew I was in trouble after that ultrasound and that cancer was exactly what they were looking for, but they didn't want me to panic, which instead left me feeling in the dark, lied to, and unable to trust that phrase from any provider without the context supporting the claim. From that day forward, "we're not worried about it" would translate to "we're very worried and just don't know how or have enough information to break the news yet."

That call hit me harder than my initial diagnosis. For the first time, I had allowed myself to have hope for the future, but the rug felt like it had just been pulled out from under me once again, this time with a much harder fall. When I was first diagnosed, I was crushed, but I still generally felt well. I didn't know how long it would last or how quickly the disease would progress, but I didn't actually "feel sick." I still had the opportunity to make the most of whatever time I had.

But now, crippled by what felt like a rather slow recovery from surgery, I actually felt sick. I still couldn't go for the long walks I enjoyed so much, couldn't play with Baxter on the floor or even enjoy a good laugh with Brian without the pain radiating throughout my body. If three new lesions had popped up in a month, what would happen after two or three months?

Without answers to those questions, I began looking for context on my own. I searched through posts in every kidney cancer Facebook group, first looking for outcomes from liver resections (of which I found only one, given the rarity of the procedure for kidney cancer), then on outcomes for liver metastases (mets) in general. I scanned through each post, mentally cataloging progression rates and the language used for each. I knew what I had was rare, so I couldn't make direct comparisons, but I could at least get the context for what was considered aggressive and what wasn't. And the context I was gathering so far wasn't easing my worries.

After making my own post and searching for advice and experiences from other patients, I moved over to a liver cancer group. I'd joined the group just before my surgery, as it was open to patients with liver mets and had lots of members who had undergone liver resections before. I'd posted a question or two before surgery asking what to expect and received great advice from a few patients who'd walked the path before. So I posted again, this time asking if anyone who'd had a liver resection had ever had a recurrence, how long after their resection it had recurred, and what the outcome or treatment had been afterward.

The responses only continued to add to my fear. There weren't many replies, and as I went back and searched through the posts in the group, most patients who had once posted questions similar to mine had since passed away, their profiles marked with tributes and memorials from loved ones on their page.

The handful of replies to my question included two early-stage liver cancer patients who'd had liver resections and no recurrence for five to ten years, and then there were several posts from caregivers whose partners had had early recurrence with aggressive disease, each of them detailing the brutal suffering their loved ones had endured before their eventual passing three to six months later. I grew nauseous as I lay in bed, picturing my own fate and wondering how much time I had left. I stared up toward the ceiling, closed my eyes, and said a silent prayer.

I might not consider myself religious, but I still pray often. I was raised Mormon, and although I left the church in my teens and never rejoined any other faiths afterward, I never gave up the act of prayer. I struggled with religion and the way I'd seen it pit good people against each other. But after I was diagnosed, all the well-intended advice to turn to God made me begin to question if my lack of faith was why this had all happened in the first place.

I tried to be a good person, help others in need, and support those around me every chance I could. I was kind, courteous, and always tried to give more than I took. But did none of that matter if it wasn't religion pushing me to do so? Was the cancer a manifestation of my lack of faith? Was it all my fault?

In the early days of my diagnosis, these questions often tortured me. So I leaned in and tried to reignite my faith, rereading scriptures and searching for answers. But I found myself even more bitter and confused than before. I struggled to see and take from religion what others did. I couldn't find the peace everyone spoke of.

Where we each find purpose and meaning in life is deeply personal. For me, that's not religion, but I wouldn't say I don't believe in something more. I don't know if I'd call it God, a higher power, or even unified energy, but I think what you call it is far less important than the impact and significance it carries. So, as I found myself grappling once again with the prospect of death, I turned to where I found peace as I closed my eyes in prayer.

Each night before surgery, I'd prayed for more time. I asked for the strength to make it through what felt like insurmountable odds. I promised if I woke up on the other side of a successful surgery, I'd use the time I'd been given to pay it forward to others. I had a deep burning passion to give back and knew that I could; I just needed the time to do it.

After making it through surgery, I thought I'd been given that time, but now I found myself confused, scared, and searching for meaning. If I was going to die anyway, why couldn't I have just gone while I was under for surgery, never waking back up? If I couldn't fulfill my promise, why did I have to suffer through the pain? I begged for answers and to understand the why and found nothing but deafening silence and a collection of tear-soaked tissues at my bedside.

Desperate for anything to blunt the fear consuming me, I decided that if all else was out of my control, maybe it was time to face the fear head on. To ask the questions I was afraid to know the answers to. What if knowing what it's like to die could teach me about how to live with the time I had?

I opened the browser on my phone and typed in one question—"What does it feel like to die from liver failure"— then proceeded to lose myself in hours of search results, videos, and hospice brochures. Do I acknowledge that it was a pretty massive leap to go from "we're not too concerned" to planning my death from liver failure? One hundred percent. But I was tired of being blindsided and paralyzed by fear anytime things didn't go as planned. I wanted to know what the finish line was like so I knew how to pace myself for the rest of the race.

For the next several hours, I leaned into the fear. At first, it felt wrong, like the act of even looking into death was a betrayal of the life I was currently living. Firsthand accounts from caregivers were traumatizing, but I noticed a clear difference in the process when a patient had hospice involved. There was often a peacefulness described in their transition to the other side, wherever or whatever the other side may be. Nothing about dying sounded peaceful to me, so I began learning more about hospice.

The more I learned, I became both comforted and curious. In a time of so much suffering, there was a sense of peace in the way people described their time in hospice, even for patients actively dying. Half the reason I was scared to die was fear of the process of dying and the pain it would bring. The other half was fear of the finality of it all. I found comfort in both the more I explored.

It was clear the process of dying was far from glamorous or perfect for anyone, but the more I learned about hospice, the more I learned it didn't have to be full of pain. The pain could be managed and mitigated, replaced with moments of comfort, tranquility, and even joy amid an inevitable farewell.

As I dove deeper, the finality of it all began to feel more distant as well. Many of the hospice resources I came across described end-of-life visions or similar experiences, labeled in different terms. The striking similarities between these experiences were impossible to ignore. They usually occurred in the final days or weeks before a patient's passing, during lucid, cognizant moments. Patients would often describe dear loved ones who'd already passed away coming to visit or to take them on a trip. As I tried to imagine myself in their shoes, these kinds of encounters sounded like the hauntings of a paranormal movie, but the patients weren't scared. Instead, they described feeling extreme peace and closure around their final days.

I found these stories and descriptions comforting, but I was also curious and skeptical. How did people from all around the world, with different backgrounds, beliefs, and cultures, end up having similar experiences? Could they all be drug-induced hallucinations? But even so, why were they all so similar, and how did they end up happening to people who even weren't medicated?

Looking for answers, I continued to dive deeper, and over the next few days I'd explore everything I could get my hands on discussing end-of-life visions and the seemingly closely related near-death experiences, everything from first-person accounts to research papers, anything I could find to explain the phenomenon.

I'm the type of person who will research something I don't understand to exhaustion until the pieces make sense. Then I flip the argument and actively try to find anything I can to disprove my findings in an effort to try to uncover as much of the full picture as I possibly can before coming to my own conclusions. Believing in end-of-life visions or near-death experiences felt a bit woo-woo to me and uncomfortable to explore, but it also aligned enough with some of my personal experiences, like the way my great-grandmother had described seeing a bright white light she was drawn to and the warmth and peace it brought her after a cardiac event. Or the peaceful, pain-free feeling I'd had after I passed out in the ICU.

I didn't feel like I'd had a near-death experience myself, but if I looked at it from that viewpoint, I wouldn't have been surprised if my great-grandma did. And what I had experienced after the incident in the ICU, the peace and calmness I felt, the absence of all pain—it all gave me a lot of hope that the end might not all be about suffering.

While these experiences and stories felt comforting, they also felt a little too mystical to believe. Surely there must be a scientific explanation for it all. So I sifted through every study I could find, looking for an explanation. Surely this must have been brought to resolution by now. However, despite the numerous hypotheses and studies, I didn't find any I felt fully accounted for or explained the profound nature of these experiences. Many of the studies even concluded that themselves, leaving me more intrigued and curious than before.

This would normally be my cue to keep digging, but before I did, I paused and asked myself what I was truly looking for. If there was a scientific explanation for it, would knowing what it was take away from the comfort of these experiences? Was I seeking validation of my fears, or solace to soothe my anxious mind? After concluding it was the latter, I gave myself permission to lean into it all—to leave this beautiful mystery unsolved. Even if I got it all wrong in the end, there was only one way I was ever going to find out. Until then, I'd let these stories bring me peace.

— 30 —

*We raised the final $5k and funded the first ever patient-led
Chromophobe kidney cancer grant! I'm filled with so many
emotions and tears of joy. Thank you, thank you, thank
you!!*
—Instagram post, August 13, 2021

A FTER I MET with my doctors to review my scans and after
the final report came in, it was determined that the new
lesions weren't technically new. It was still too soon after surgery to know exactly what they were, but they appeared to be
residual disease, not new lesions.

I felt instant relief but also felt worried about what might
happen to the spots in the coming months while I was off
treatment and we waited to rescan. But the news eased up the
fear that had consumed me the previous few days and allowed
me to reframe my thinking. If I couldn't control the outcome
between now and then, what could I control? Where could I
place my time instead of spiraling in bed? This existential cri-
sis I'd been in led me to ask myself, *If tomorrow isn't promised,
what would I wish I'd done today?*

This wasn't an easy mentality to shift to. My whole life,
I'd set arbitrary milestones and ambiguous goals I expected
myself to hit before indulging in things I viewed as a luxury or
reward. You don't buy the dream car until you'd "made it"—
whatever "it" was. No taking chances without a safety net, and
don't blindly pursue passion without a plan. My life had been

so meticulously and carefully planned before cancer, setting me up for a future that I had no guarantee I'd see.

However, now with a shifted perspective, anytime I justified inaction with a "I'll do it when . . . ," I pushed back and challenged myself, asking, *If tomorrow isn't promised, will I regret not doing it today?* Unsurprisingly, the answer to that question was almost always a resounding yes. If I truly wanted to live whatever time I had left to the fullest, like I'd promised myself I would, I'd better stop waiting for the right moments and start creating them instead.

The first time I put this into practice was when I saw that the grant I'd been fundraising for with a group of other patients, the one I'd fundraised toward for my birthday, was only $5,000 away from completion. I remembered thinking, *As soon as I feel better, I'll start fundraising again; maybe I'll hold a 5k.* Then suddenly, I paused, remembering the promise I'd made to myself, and I asked, *If I never feel better than I do today, would I regret not doing it now?*

The chromophobe RCC grant funding felt so deeply personal to me. Since my diagnosis, the five other women I'd been fundraising for it with had become like family. We'd grown so close over our shared experiences and our desire to bring this grant to life that it was at the top of my list of things I wanted to stick around for, to watch succeed. Immediately, I knew the answer to that question. If it wasn't promised I'd feel better tomorrow, I'd regret not starting today. I jumped onto Facebook and threw together a fundraiser, a 5k for the last $5K.

Barely a month out of surgery, while still not able to walk over a quarter of a mile on my own in the heat, I was pledging to complete a 5k. While I certainly wouldn't be running it, in just four weeks, on the two-month anniversary of my surgery, I'd promise to walk 3.1 miles to bring in the final funding for the grant. Was the timing ideal? Absolutely not. And was it going to be hard? No doubt. But time and the future were a luxury not promised. If it was important for me to see this thing through to completion, I was going to have to make the moment, not wait for it.

As a group, we rallied together and made it happen. On August 29, 2021, I held a virtual 5k, honoring the promise I'd made, and friends, family, and loved ones helped us bring in the final funding for the grant. I may have moved at a turtle's pace, but I proudly walked out every last step of that 3.1 miles. And I don't know if I've ever been prouder in my life, not only of myself but of the sheer determination and resolve of the other women in our group. This wasn't just a fundraiser; this was setting the stage for change. For a rare cancer and a group of patients often left behind, this would be a catalyst for hope.

After recognizing the joy and fulfillment this experience brought, I rolled the same mindset into nearly every aspect of my life. Instead of waiting for tomorrow, I began capital-izing on today. I bought my dream car and had it wrapped in a design in honor of Andrew and Driven to Cure, something that would serve as a reminder to me, every day, to live in the moment. And instead of waiting until I had recovered, knew how to edit videos, and even had a proper camera, I started making more content online, sharing my experiences for oth-ers and creating the resources I'd gone looking for but couldn't find when I was diagnosed.

I even built an app to help patients with providers at sev-eral different institutions manage their care. I published and wrapped it up literally as I was being admitted to the hospital for a follow-up procedure. I was able to do and accomplish so much more in the two months I spent awaiting my scans after surgery than I had in nearly the entire year prior. I'd traded the fear of death for an addiction to life, and I wanted to make the most out of every second of it.

This newfound zest for life didn't come without its moments of despair. When we rescanned in October to check the few lesions we were watching, we found out that they were indeed tumors that'd been left behind and that they were still growing. After receiving the news, I was crushed and I cried the entire night. But the difference this time around was that I didn't let the fear destroy me, I let it motivate me. It increased my urgency and made me push harder to ensure I accomplished all that I'd set out to do within whatever block of certainty I still had in my control. Which meant pushing the app that I'd created and taking care of final bug fixes while I was literally being admitted to the NIH, awaiting an ablation procedure to have tumors burned from my liver the next morning—for no other reason than because I wanted it to exist in the world.

I pushed hard up to the procedure, knowing the window within my control would be closing soon. Then I coasted through with no plans or expectations on myself while I made it through recovery—where my unoccupied mind most certainly opened me up to more worry in the hospital. I greatly appreciated Brian, who'd stop by to visit, and the nurses, who helped me pass the time by offering a much-needed distraction. Including my favorite nurse from that stay, who after checking on her other patients would come keep me company and chat with me at night when I couldn't sleep.

This new cadence of packing in every ounce of life I could until the next scans or procedure, then riding out the window of unknowns, would soon become a familiar and steady rhythm, my constant in all the uncertainty.

— 31 —

It took facing death for me to learn to live life to the fullest.

I LEFT MY PROCEDURE with the hope that my next set of scans would come back with no evidence of disease. Every morning, I looked to a photo of a bell I'd taped to my mirror and pictured the triumphant finish line. So after surgery, when my scans didn't come back clear, it was crushing, but I was still hopeful a celebration might be just around the corner after the second procedure, the ablations, took care of the rest of the disease. But unfortunately, I'd soon learn the end of treatment was more like a moving target than something that could be tied up neatly in a bow.

My next set of scans after the ablations showed that destruction of the targeted lesions had been successful, but they still noted a few small residual spots. They were all under five millimeters and too small to characterize but were suspicious for metastatic disease, with recommended close follow-up on the subsequent scans. As I read the report, I was grateful the procedure was successful and that there were no new lesions, but if I was being honest, I also felt a bit robbed.

Society had built up the image and narrative of battling cancer in my mind as something with clear defining moments of victory and defeat. And although I'd learned enough to know better at this point, there was still a small piece of me holding out hope. When I was first diagnosed, on my most difficult days I'd often seek out videos of patients ringing the bell, surrounded by their loved ones. Tears of joy would stream down my face as I played them on a loop, celebrating their win and hoping to experience one of my own one day.

I had such a conflicted relationship with that bell. I could still feel the jealousy, guilt, and sadness I'd tried to suppress when I'd heard it ring out in the background in the early days. It brought a whirlwind of emotion, the immense joy of celebrating with others contrasting with the stark reminder that treatment goals for me weren't curative. Perhaps that's partly why I became so attached to it, seeing it as a symbol of something that felt so unattainable. It was the marker of a hard-fought battle, one I wasn't expected to win.

But it also symbolized far more than the celebration and cheering it elicited. It felt like permission. Permission to close a painful and grueling chapter, to let go of the fear, and to start living again. Everyone around me seemed to think I was out of the woods. Doctors encouraged me to celebrate the win and to get back to life. But without closure and definitive answers, I didn't know how. So instead of getting back to the life I had, I started to craft a new one.

With life and certainly only ever guaranteed for three months at a time, I set out to make as much of an impact as I could between each scan cycle. I thought about quitting my job so I could spend more of my time focused on the things that were important to me. But I quickly realized insurance was one of those important things, so I scaled back to part-time instead.

I spent the rest of my time creating content to help other patients learn about their disease, advocating for kidney and rare cancers, and building out my app. I'd go for long walks around the park, often sprinting through the back segments, simply to feel the wind on my face. I was out of breath and

out of shape, something that before would have sparked negative thoughts or emotions. However, now, as I gasped for air, I
found myself lost in the beauty of feeling my lungs expand and
my body recover. Remembering what it was like to think I'd
never feel these things again reminded me of what a privilege
it was to do so. One I'd been given, at least in part, by a man
who was now losing the very same abilities I was regaining.

Just a week after my scans in October had uncovered
the residual tumors we'd have to ablate, Bruce went for his
annual scans at the NIH. He had the same mutation Andrew
did, which carried a higher risk for kidney cancer, so he was
scanned annually to keep a close eye on things. The night
he received his results, he sent me an email with the report,
and my stomach sank. He hadn't met with the team yet, but I
knew: this was cancer.

A week later when it was confirmed, my heart shattered into
a million pieces. Not only did he have cancer, but it was pan-
creatic cancer, one of the most aggressive types. The news hit
hard. How could someone who'd given and done so much for
others find themselves here? Just a few months ago, I was the one
who was facing an inoperable cancer and a bleak prognosis, but
now we'd swapped places. The very same surgeon who'd taken
a chance on me was now breaking the news to him that surgery
wouldn't be a viable option. But Bruce's motto, inherited from
Andrew, was to never, ever, ever give up. So he pushed on.

As I was recovering in the hospital from my ablations,
Bruce had an appointment of his own there and came to visit
me afterward. He sat back in the chair across from the bed
and updated me on the HLRCC patients he'd connected with
through Driven to Cure that he was so excited to hear were
doing well. He was fighting a battle of his own but still not skip-
ping a beat in the celebration of others. He'd chosen to keep
his diagnosis private at the time, and although we'd messaged
about it often, I could tell he didn't want to talk about it at the
hospital. So we made small talk instead and chatted about

Driven to Cure before it was time for him to leave. Before we said our goodbyes, I thanked him one more time and promised him if he ever needed me for anything, I'd be here for him, just as he had been there for me. He silently nodded, and both our eyes filled with tears before he cut through heaviness in the room with a joke about me making him cry as he stood up to leave. We'd stay in close contact over the next year, but that day would be the last time we saw each other in person.

Over the next two years, I'd lose many friends to cancer, something that never gets easier with time. But the passing of both Bruce and McKinley Grace (MG) were two losses that truly crushed me. Bruce passed in December 2022 just before Christmas and MG that following February 2023, two weeks after Brian and I returned from Bruce's funeral service. The two of them were my constants and my support system through my darkest days. I struggled to reconcile how they could be gone while I was still here.

I learned of MG's passing while I was at a writers' conference, pitching this very book. It happened to be a mile down the street from the largest oncology conference for kidney cancer the same weekend, so I'd bought tickets to both. I knew MG hadn't been doing well; she'd joined one of my TikTok lives a couple weeks prior from the ER. Lives often feel like a one-way street, so with four hundred people on the live, we didn't get to converse much, but I was able to send her well wishes. And as I described her to those tuning in, I showed them the ring I'd made with the words YOU CAN stamped into it, matching the sign she'd sent and the encouragement she'd given just before surgery. It was my reminder that I can do hard things. I took it off as I held it up to the camera, and I told her it was my turn to send that encouragement back her way and that I'd continue praying for her. She replied with a final comment, thanking me and letting me know my friendship meant the world to her, a sentiment that instantly brought me to tears and that I echoed right back before she signed off.

Over the next week, things had taken a turn for the worse, but I kept praying her body would recover and she'd pull through. Unfortunately, things didn't improve and I learned of her passing while I was in San Francisco after the first day of the conference. I cried the entire night and woke the next morning with my eyes nearly swollen shut. Devastated and unsure of how to continue, I considered flying home early. I didn't know how to continue with her gone and didn't think I could make it through the day without the tears. But one of the major bonds and commonalities we shared was our desire to see better treatments and improvements for rare kidney cancers. MG herself had even had dreams of going into oncology or research one day. I knew she would want me at the conference.

I didn't know how I'd find the strength and wasn't sure I was doing the right thing, so with tears streaming down my face, I paused, and with desperation, I prayed. I was upset that I kept losing so many friends—so many people I felt deserved to be here more than I did. I needed something to tell me there was more to this world than the suffering and pain I kept witnessing.

Praying out loud as if MG could hear me, I told her I knew she'd want me there but I didn't know how I was going to find the strength to get through the day or even if I should. I needed to know she was okay and that going to the conference was the right thing to do. I asked for a sign, one so obvious I wouldn't be able to dismiss it. Then I picked a random object. If I came across something with flowers, that would be my sign.

It was a few days past valentines day and I was in the middle of the city. So they felt like a pretty safe bet. If flowers somehow crossed my path in an obvious way that day, I would take it as my sign. I twisted the ring at my finger, paused, took a deep breath, and headed out the door.

I managed to make it through the conference with only two breakdowns, one when another patient advocate passed along condolences and another when MG's father called to ask me if I'd like to record a video, to speak at her celebration of life. I was truly touched and honored he'd asked, not only because of the close friendship MG and I had shared but also because her father had asked me to announce that a cell line from MG's cancer was being made to help further research for other patients one day—something I knew was both deeply important to her and the reason I was actually at this convention; I was here to talk to researchers about this very thing for other rare kidney cancers. It was the confirmation I needed to remind me that this was exactly where MG would have wanted me to be.

As the day wrapped up, I headed back to my hotel, where the writers' conference was taking place. Both physically and emotionally exhausted, I planned to just head straight back up to the room. But feeling a bit guilty for missing the entire day, I decided to check what the final session was in the room just a few steps away from the elevator. It was a session on audiobooks, one I'd earmarked to attend. I chose to step in and listen from the back of the room, knowing I could easily step back out if it became too much.

It was a good session, but I admittedly was distracted through half of it. Zoned out, I was caught by surprise when it came to a close and the woman next to me struck up a conversation about how great it was. I nodded my head and played along, echoing back the only few words I'd caught so I didn't give away the fact that I'd missed half the session.

As we were chatting, I noticed an older gentleman I'd had a conversation with the day before making his way around the room. He'd been in the industry for over forty years and was offering free consulting to writers at the conference. I'd wanted his advice but had been too intimidated to ask until I bumped into him as I was lost and looking for a session the day before. I hadn't been wearing my glasses, so I'd squinted in his general direction trying to read the board behind him, which had resulted in him asking if I was looking for him and wanted a consultation. Too embarrassed to tell him I'd actually been trying to look at the board behind him, I rolled with it and told him I was.

He invited me to pull up a seat next to him and asked what he could help with. Completely unprepared, I gave him the CliffsNotes of my story—told him about my diagnosis, how I'd decided to write a memoir about my experience to raise money for research but that I'd never written anything before and didn't know where to begin or honestly even if my writing was trash. He was so kind and moved by my story that anytime we'd crossed paths afterward, he'd introduced me to whoever he was with as "one of the most inspiring people he'd ever met," which would instantly flush my cheeks with embarrassment. But I also appreciated the acknowledgment, since I was too scared to talk to anyone on my own.

I'd come in late, so we didn't chat in the audiobook session, but while I was talking with the woman next to me after it ended, I caught the older gentleman's bright-red top hat out of the corner of my eye as he made his way to the front of the room. A few moments later, he very briefly popped into our conversation to hand me something, simply stating, "I feel like you could use this," as he handed me a card and swiftly stepped away. The woman and I looked at each other, confused, as I looked down at what he'd handed me. Sitting just over top of MG's ring as I grasped the card in my hand was a packet of Shasta daisy seeds. The business card for the voice actress presenting in the sessions was a literal packet of flower seeds—beautiful white-and-yellow daisies on the front, her name, email, and website on the back.

My eyes filled with tears, and I frantically looked up, trying to place the man in the room to ask why he'd handed me the card, but he'd already gone. If I was looking for a sign, this was sure going to be hard to ignore.

Losing so many friends from cancer has been one of the most difficult parts of the journey, but it's also been one that's taught me the most about life. It has shown me how fragile life is and how quickly things can turn. It's taught me how to live in the moment and make the most of the good days; to never miss an opportunity to tell someone how much they mean to me and that our impact on the world doesn't end when we leave it. Let the ripples we leave behind become powerful currents to guide others on their path.

After my ablations, I might not have had any more certainty in my future. I didn't have a cancer-free declaration I could share with family and friends or any more answers than we did before, but what I did have was more time. So, while I could, I made the most of it.

I got more done in those three months than I'd ever thought possible and found myself genuinely happy and truly excited about life. Brian and I traveled to see family and friends, I created tools and resources for other patients, and I gave back as much as I could. Things were going so well that Brian and I even began planning for our future, a new addition to our little family. This little fur-covered bundle, with tiny paws and short little legs, might have looked a bit different than the family we'd planned in the past, but the tiny kitten we brought home after my next scans would be the newest member of our family and loved just the same.

With each new scan I received, I still hadn't made it to NED. Those small lesions in my liver were always mentioned, but they were stable, which bought me more time off treatment to make it to the next scan. Another three months. Over this period, I started a YouTube channel to create the videos I'd gone looking for when I was diagnosed. I fundraised and traveled. I spent the first anniversary of my surgery hiking through Zion National Park with two of my cancer buddies I'd met online, celebrating the fact that we were spending time on mountain cliffs instead of operating tables. Brian and

I finally bought a house, and I even got a new job closer to health care.

I finally learned that I didn't need a shiny bell to ring for permission to live life. That there is just as much celebration in the journey as there is in the milestones. Learning to live with cancer, to make the most out of each and every single day, has taught me far more about life than the symbolic ringing of a bell ever could. It's not about making it to the finish line, it's about cherishing the race. It's feeling the wind on your face and the air in your lungs. It's recognizing your strength through the pain and beauty in the recovery.

After nearly a year and a half of three-month intervals after surgery, I finally received my very first NED, one that I tried to fish out of Dr. Msaouel before those beautiful words ever officially landed in my report. It was far more anticlimactic than I'd ever anticipated after I'd envisioned the moment a million times before. There was no bell, no clapping, no cheering, just Dr. Msaouel and me in a room after another long stream of my never-ending questions, ending on, "So it's been a year of stability. What do we call me at this point?" And him confirming that, although we didn't know what the spots in my liver were, with over a year off treatment and without any growth, he felt comfortable calling me NED. I tried to suppress my excitement, as my attachment to those words felt a little unwarranted. I mean, nothing had technically changed—but this was still a win.

"I like the sound of that," I said, grinning ear to ear.

He chuckled softly while I knocked on the closest piece of wood I could find. "Me too," he replied, knocking back.

No evidence of disease is really just four words to describe a snapshot in time. There's no promise and no guarantee. Yet hearing those words—after being told it was something I'd likely never reach—still felt like a triumph against the odds. I walked out of my appointment, called the elevator, and made it down to the lobby just like I had every time before. I looked around at all the beautiful faces surrounding me, the strangers embarking on their own battles, patients who I knew would give anything to trade places with me right now. This moment felt like it was worth documenting or celebrating in some way, but in a room full of other patients still in the thick of their fight, it didn't feel right.

I walked out to sit by the fountain just outside the building, the one I'd walked past a million times before as I reflected on how far I'd come. When we were at MD Anderson for our first appointment, I remembered how I'd made Brian slow down and pause at this fountain as we walked by it, partially to take in its beauty but also as a stalling tactic, knowing I was only a few hundred feet away from where we'd have to part ways and I'd be forced to face my fate alone. I wished he were here to share this moment.

I felt a gentle mist of rain begin. If I wanted to document this with a photo, I'd better get it now before everyone took cover. I stopped the closest passerby and asked them to snap a picture of me in front of the sign just before the gentle misting turned into a sheet of rain.

My phone began pinging with severe-weather alerts and flood advisories. With my car's battery already on empty, I knew I had to make it to the chargers before the heart of the storm hit, as I wouldn't have enough charge to afford any road closures or detours. So I quickly made it to the car and hit the road.

The rain poured down, blurring the world beyond my windshield, as my wipers struggled to keep up. I'd driven through Texas storms before, but the sheer amount of rainfall coming down with this one was astounding. The roads were filling and the drains struggling to keep up by the time I finally pulled into the parking lot. At least I'd made it; I could wait out the rest from here.

I plugged in the car with a constant wipe of my brow to keep the rain out of my eyes, then quickly sought shelter back in the driver's seat. With my clothes soaked and shoes squishy, I let out a hearty laugh. *Well, not quite how I saw today going, but man, how cool is it I'm here for this. I didn't think I'd still be alive, but here I am. I may be squishy and wet from a torrential downpour, but hey, at least I'm even here to be squishy and wet.* I shook my head as I laughed in disbelief, bewildered by it all. *Life's crazy.*

I heard my stomach grumble. It was four PM and I hadn't eaten anything all day. So while the car charged, I decided to run into the store to grab a few snacks for the road. I walked back out with two Smart Waters, almonds, and an impulse buy of a fifty-cent mini bag of Cheetos, breakfast of champions. The storm still raging on, I started sprinting back to the car before realizing the splash of running through the puddles beneath me was getting me just as wet as the rain was above. I slowed to a walk, closed my eyes, and laughed as I tilted my head back up toward the sky, taking in the moment instead of rushing through it.

As I lowered my head back down and opened my eyes, I saw a man with a bike approaching from a distance. He was wearing a white shirt that was now stretched and translucent, soaked from the storm, with cargo shorts and a ratty pair of sneakers. He wheeled his bike over as he cautiously approached, apologizing profusely and trying to ensure I didn't feel threatened. "I'm so sorry, ma'am. I know I should never approach a woman. But I was trying to make it downtown for services before this storm hit. I'm hungry but won't be able to make it down before they close. I hate to ask this, but do you have any food to share?"

Caught a bit off guard, I looked down at the bag of snacks in my hand as I tried to process and analyze the situation.

"I'm not looking for money, I'm just hungry," he said softly before looking down at the contents of my bag and apologizing, "but it doesn't look like you've got much; I'm so sorry—I shouldn't have asked."

I could give him those Cheetos I'd impulse-bought at the register; *I don't need to eat them anyways*, I thought. But that didn't exactly seem like much. I looked up at him as he started to back away. "I don't have much in the bag, but there's a café right there. If you follow me over, I could buy you a meal," I offered up as I pointed to a café on the corner, just under a quarter mile away.

"That sounds amazing, but . . . it's raining. Are you going to go on foot?" he asked, his voice tinged with guilt for taking me up on something so far out of the way.

"Yeah, why not? I'm already wet; a little more rain won't make much of a difference. My car needs to charge anyway," I insisted as I gestured toward the café.

We both looked at each other briefly, likely both thinking, *Is this really happening?* A woman walking alone with a strange man who'd just approached her to the café down the road sounded like it was straight out of a true-crime episode. I could see the headlines now. But I didn't feel threatened by this man and could tell he could use a little help.

He turned his bike around, placing it between us as we started walking toward the cafe. Without a word, I could sense his gratitude as I watched him search for how he could provide something in return. "Okay, if you're walking, then I'll protect you," he said as he straightened up his shoulders and puffed out his chest. We both nervously laughed at the irony.

As we walked, he thanked me profusely, but I assured him it wasn't necessary. I told him I'd gotten some pretty good news and I was happy to pay it forward to make someone else's day better. He asked about my good news, then about my story. I shared with him the CliffsNotes—that I had been diagnosed with cancer a couple years ago and didn't have a great prognosis, that I'd been given a second chance by a pretty large surgery last summer, and that today I'd finally gotten to hear the words "no evidence of disease" for the very first time, something I'd never thought I'd hear.

His eyes widened and his jaw dropped. "What? I'm walking next to a miracle!" he proclaimed. "Oh my god, you kicked cancer's ass!" His excitement was more palpable than mine, as he'd now added number-one hype man alongside bodyguard to his title as we continued along our path.

"I mean, it's still cancer, so we never really know," I said humbly. "But yes, I am pretty excited about it."

The rest of the walk, as our shoes squished audibly with every step, he peppered me with questions about what it was like to have cancer, about treatment, and any pearls of wisdom I'd taken away. I squeezed in answering as much as I could on our short journey until we arrived at our destination. Upon our arrival, I went in to order, and he waited at a table outside.

Drenched, with my makeup smeared and my hair soaked, I got a crusty look from the woman at the counter, but honestly, I didn't mind; there were worse things to be judged for.

The food came out just as the rain began to let up. I filled the bag with a bunch of napkins and utensils before bringing it back out to the man. "Here you go. I hope you make it downtown safely," I said as I handed him the bag.

With a humble nod of his head, he pressed his hands together in a gesture of gratitude as he again thanked me profusely.

As I left him behind to eat and started to make my way back to the car, I assured him again that no thanks were necessary but suggested that the next chance he had to pay it forward to someone else, he could too. He promised he would as the distance between us widened and he called out, "I'll never forget you, Katie! The girl who made cancer her bitch!"

I chuckled at his candidness as I awkwardly thanked him and waved farewell.

I laughed to myself the whole way back—at his comment, at the recklessness I'd just shown, and at how completely and utterly drenched I was. But I couldn't say I regretted it; what an experience. As I got back to the car, it was fully charged, and as

I went to unplug it, I looked up and caught a full rainbow cast off in the distance. My eyes instantly filled with tears. There was no way this was real life. What a beautiful endcap to the most incredible day.

After all the time I'd spent daydreaming over what it'd be like to reach no evidence of disease or to ring that bell, I'd never imagined the moment would look anything like this. Or that the first person I'd celebrate with would be a man experiencing homelessness, drenched in a Walmart parking lot. But now that I'd found myself here, I wouldn't have it any other way. Life is unpredictable, it's messy, and it doesn't always go according to plan, but finding the beauty in between is what life is all about. So make the most out of every single day. Take chances and don't be afraid of failure. If you can't find the moments, make them. And never let the fear of tomorrow rob you of the joy of today.

Being diagnosed with cancer was the hardest thing I've ever gone through. But it also allowed me to live more fully than I ever thought was possible. If I have one final piece of advice or parting words of wisdom I hope you take from my story, it's that I wish everyone could experience the joy I've been blessed with in the past few years. It took facing death for me to learn to live life to the fullest. Do me a favor and don't follow in my footsteps. Find meaning in today, and if all else fails, let this book be your motivation to live life refocused.

Acknowledgments

T HE NIGHT I received my biopsy results, confirming stage four cancer, I shared on Instagram: As long as I'm still writing the story, this isn't how my story ends. At the time, I never in my wildest dreams could have imagined writing a memoir one day. Yet here we are, and it's time to extend my deepest thanks to those who've played a pivotal role in changing my tides and improving my outcome.

First and foremost, I have to express my immense gratitude to my remarkable husband, Brian. His unwavering support through every challenge we faced and his patience during our nightly "story time" sessions, as I pored over every written word, revision, and edit of these pages, has been invaluable. Brian, you are the best partner I could ever ask for, and I love you endlessly.

To my doctors and care team, without you, I wouldn't have a story to share. Thank you for not only the time you've given me but also the life and purpose you gifted me with in the process. I will forever be grateful for the chance you took on me and the many ways you have continued to support me through the years. Words will never be able to properly convey my gratitude for you.

My parents, family, and friends, thank you for rallying around me during my darkest times and for being there to support me both at home and from afar.

To the cancer community, especially those within the kidney cancer space, your guidance, support, and solidarity have been my beacon of hope. Without you, I can't imagine where I'd be.

To Catherine, Kayla, Annamaria, Melissa, Tracy, and Laura, your steadfast presence and support have been my anchor through my most difficult days. I wouldn't have become the advocate I am today without you ladies.

A heartfelt thank-you to my incredible agent, Rachel Sussman, and my editor, Laura Apperson, for believing in me and this memoir. Your countless hours of dedication have shaped this memoir into what it is today. Without you, this dream would not have become a reality.

This book is dedicated to the many patients who have supported me and the physicians who have immeasurably changed my life. While I'm unable to name everyone without turning this into a novel of its own, I must acknowledge Dr. Hernandez, Dr. Ball, Dr. Msaouel, Dr. Linehan, Dr. Kalsi, and Dr. Yorio for their exceptional care.

Lastly, to Bruce, MG, Judith, Michael, Kelly, Daniel, Patricia, and Amanda: thank you for blessing me with your friendship and support. I miss our conversations, and I will forever carry your memories with me. Our impact on the world doesn't end when we leave it. I promise to do my best to carry your legacies with me and to extend the ripple from each of your stories as we together build waves of change for better outcomes for those affected by cancer.